# THE NURSE AND
# THE DEVELOPMENTALLY
# DISABLED ADOLESCENT

# THE NURSE AND THE DEVELOPMENTALLY DISABLED ADOLESCENT

Edited by

## Mary Lou de Leon Siantz, R.N., M.N.

Director, Division of Nursing
University Affiliated Program
 for Child Development
Georgetown University Hospital

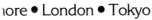

versity Park Press
nore • London • Tokyo

**UNIVERSITY PARK PRESS**
International Publishers in Science and Medicine
Chamber of Commerce Building
Baltimore, Maryland 21202

Typeset by American Graphic Arts Corporation
Manufactured in the United States of America by Universal Lithographers,
Inc., and The Optic Bindery Incorporated

**Library of Congress Cataloging in Publication Data:**
Main entry under title:

The nurse and the developmentally disabled adolescent.

Includes index.
1. Handicapped youth.   2. Pediatric nursing.
3. Child development deviations—Nursing.
I. Siantz, Mary Lou de Leon.   [DNLM:   1. Child
development deviations—Nursing texts.
2. Adolescence—Nursing texts.   3. Handicapped—
Nursing tests.   4. Rehabilitation—Nursing texts. WY160 N968]
RJ138.N8      610.73´6      77-7201
ISBN 0-8391-1131-2

# CONTENTS

Preface        vii
Contributors        ix
Consulting Editors        xi
Acknowledgments        xiii

chapter one
INTRODUCTION / *Mary Lou de Leon Siantz, R.N., M.N.*        1
chapter two
NURSES' RESPONSIBILITY IN ADOLESCENCE / ———
*Mary Lou de Leon Siantz, R.N., M.N., and*
*Jennie Downer Austin, R.N., B.S.*        17
chapter three
PHYSICAL DEVELOPMENT / *Richard Jones, M.D.*        49
chapter four
PSYCHOLOGICAL CONCEPTS / *Kathy S. Katz, Ph.D.*        61
chapter five
THE ADOLESCENT AND THE FAMILY /
*Inta Adamovics Rutins, M.S.W., ACSW*        75
chapter six
THE ADOLESCENT IN THE COMMUNITY /
*Virginia Williams, M.A.*        91
chapter seven
SPECIAL EDUCATION NEEDS / *Michael Bender, Ed.D.*        103
chapter eight
DENTAL NEEDS / *Beverly A. Entwistle, R.D.H., M.P.H.*        119
chapter nine
NUTRITION AND NUTRITION EDUCATION NEEDS /
*Mary Helen Greenwood, R.D., M.S.*        139
chapter ten
VOCATIONAL NEEDS / *Kevin P. Lynch, Ph.D.*        173
chapter eleven
SEX EDUCATION / *Vivian Dee, R.N., M.N.*        187
chapter twelve
THE PATH TO ADULTHOOD: Adolescence, Disability, and the
Law / *Bertram Robert Cottine, J.D.*        213
chapter thirteen
TOMORROW: Toward Fulfillment as an Adult /
*Ann M. Zuzich, R.N., M.S.*        233

Index        245

# PREFACE

This book provides an integrated and comprehensive approach for identifying, planning, and managing the problems of developmentally disabled adolescents. It addresses problems that nurses and other health care professionals encounter as they attempt to help the developmentally disabled develop to their fullest potential and become viable members of their communities.

A growing awareness and commitment to improve the quality of life for these individuals have increased during the last decade. These people have become increasingly visible in a variety of clinical and community settings. The need for effective intervention from a variety of resources has also grown. For nurses and other health care professionals this has meant a need to increase collaboration and effective communication among disciplines that practice with this population. It has also become particularly important to understand the vocabulary, style, and approach of the various disciplines important to the adolescent period.

The growing body of literature in some of the disciplines concerned with the adolescent has been primarily directed to the members of each particular discipline. This makes it difficult for professionals outside the discipline to research specific questions. Also, little has been documented in the nursing literature that deals exclusively with the developmentally disabled as an active adolescent and potential adult, particularly the knowledge, skills, and alternative approaches the nurse must consider with this group.

This book is designed in response to these concerns. It is directed to the nurse clinician, educator, administrator, student, and other professionals working with developmentally disabled adolescents. It provides an available reference and guideline to the multiple areas, disciplines, and resources that must be considered during the adolescent period. Each chapter provides a bibliography and suggested readings for those who wish to further explore specific areas.

# CONTRIBUTORS

**Jennie Downer Austin, R.N., B.S.,** Formerly: Home Service Director, United Cerebral Palsy, Nassau County, Long Island, New York; Currently: enrolled Family-Child Nursing, Catholic University of America, Washington, D.C.

**Michael Bender, Ed.D.,** Director of Special Education, John F. Kennedy Institute for the Habilitation of Handicapped Children; Assistant Professor of Education, John Hopkins University, Baltimore, Maryland

**Bertram Robert Cottine, J.D.,** Adjunct Professor of Law, Georgetown University Law Center, Washington, D.C.

**Vivian Dee, R.N., M.N.,** Director of Nursing, Mental Retardation Program and Child Psychiatry, Neuropsychiatric Institute; Assistant Clinical Professor, Psychiatric and Community Mental Health Nursing, School of Nursing, University of California, Los Angeles, California

**Beverly A. Entwistle, R.D.H., M.P.H.,** Instructional Associate, Dental Hygiene, Institute for the Study of Mental Retardation and Related Disabilities, University of Michigan, Ann Arbor, Michigan

**Mary Helen Greenwood, R.D., M.S.,** Nutritionist, Child Development Mental Retardation Center, University of Washington, Seattle, Washington

**Richard Jones, M.D.,** Fellow Adolescent Medicine, Division of Adolescent Medicine, Department of Pediatrics, Georgetown University, Washington, D.C.

**Kathy S. Katz, Ph.D.,** Staff Psychologist, University Affiliated Program for Child Development; Assistant Professor, Department of Pediatrics, School of Medicine, Georgetown University, Washington, D.C.

**Kevin P. Lynch, Ph.D.,** Associate Research Scientist, Vocational Services Component, Institute for the Study of Mental Retardation and Related Disabilities, University of Michigan, Ann Arbor, Michigan

**Inta Adamovics Rutins, M.S.W., ACSW,** Staff Social Worker, Adolescent Team, Intensive Care Unit, Psychiatric Institute, Washington, D.C.; Formerly: Instructor, Department of Pediatrics, University Affiliated Program for Child Development, Georgetown University; Assistant Professor, Howard University School of Social Work, Washington, D.C.

**Mary Lou de Leon Siantz, R.N., M.N.,** Director, Division of Nursing, University Affiliated Program for Child Development; Instructor, Department of Pediatrics, School of Medicine, Georgetown University; Instructor, School of Nursing, Georgetown University, Adjunct Assistant Professor, School of Nursing, Catholic University of America, Washington, D.C.

**Virginia Williams, M.A.**, Associate Director for Community Services, University Affiliated Program for Child Development, Georgetown University; Instructor, Department of Pediatrics, School of Medicine, Georgetown, University, Washington, D.C.

**Ann M. Zuzich, R.N., M.S.**, Associate Professor, Department of Psychiatric Mental Health Nursing, School of Nursing, Wayne State University, Detroit, Michigan

# CONSULTING EDITORS

**Jasper Harvey, Ph.D.,** Office of Education, Bureau for the Education of the Handicapped; Director, Division of Personnel Preparation (Chapter 7)

**Betty Lucas, M.P.H.,** Staff Nutritionist, Child Development and Mental Retardation Center, University of Washington (Chapter 9)

**Phyllis Magrab, Ph.D.,** Associate Professor, Department of Pediatrics; Director, University Affiliated Program for Child Development, Georgetown University (Chapters 4 and 6)

**Arthur Nowak, M.A., D.M.D.,** Associate Professor, College Dentistry, University of Iowa (Chapter 8)

**Jane Rees, M.S.,** Staff Nutritionist, Child Development and Mental Retardation Center, University of Washington (Chapter 9)

**Robert Shearin, M.D.,** Clinical Assistant Professor, Department of Pediatrics, Adolescent Medicine, Georgetown University Hospital

**James E. Siantz, Ph.D.,** Office of Education, Bureau for the Education of the Handicapped; Project Officer, Division of Personnel Preparation

# ACKNOWLEDGMENTS

Special appreciation is extended to my husband, James E. Siantz, for his support, assistance, and encouragement throughout the production of this book. Special thanks go to Dr. Phyllis Magrab, Director of the University Affiliated Program for Child Development, Georgetown University, for her support, and to Dr. Jasper Harvey for his special help with resources. I am particularly indebted to the competence and diligence of Ms. Debra Friedman. Special thanks are also due the staff of the University Affiliated Program for Child Development for their patience and support. Finally, special thanks go to Vivian and Mrs. P. for helping to identify the need for such a book.

Illustrations in Chapter II were done by Lynn Mancini.
Photographs in Chapter II were done by Jackie Feiner.
Photographs in Chapter IX were done by Jan Smyth

*To Jim*

# chapter one

# INTRODUCTION

## Mary Lou de Leon Siantz, R.N., M.N.

Adolescence, the period ranging from as early as 10 to as late as 21, is a time when emancipation from the primary family unit is one of the central developmental tasks. During this period, an individual must also develop: 1) a personal identity, 2) a sexual role, and 3) the ability to make certain vocational choices (Hammar and Barnard, 1966). If the adolescent has a developmental disability he* faces additional problems. A developmental disability may be attributable to: 1) mental retardation, 2) cerebral palsy, 3) epilepsy, 4) autism, 5) dyslexia, or 6) any other conditions closely related to mental retardation that result in intellectual and adaptive impairment. It originates before age 18, may continue indefinitely, and constitutes a substantial handicap (HEW, 1975). Although an adolescent with a developmental disability may have the physical attributes of a normal adolescent, he may not always possess the ability to cope with the awesome responsibility of preparing for vocational competence and to develop the social and emotional characteristics that will enable him to gain social acceptance (Chinn, Drew, Logan, 1975).

For parents, the onset of pubertal change with its emerging sexuality can often become a potent catalyst. Adolescence may precipitate a family crisis and provide a strong impetus for seeking help. As parents themselves grow older, they become increasingly concerned over who will take the responsibility of caring for their developmentally disabled child.

Yet it is during this period that special programs, services, and institutional concern for the developmentally disabled begin to rapidly drop off. Local communities lack prepared personnel, vocational training, resources, social or recreational activities, and residential

---

* Gender-specific pronouns are used for purposes of clarity only. They are not meant to be exclusionary.

facilities for the developmentally disabled adolescent. Health care professionals may overlook the need for the ongoing management and periodic re-evaluation critical to the maximal independence the adolescent may achieve at home, with family, peers, at work, and in the community. Communication and coordination with the school also diminishes (Stedman, 1971). Problems the adolescent and his family might have are frequently resolved on a crisis basis rather than prevented.

Health care professionals may feel at a loss as to how to help the adolescent and his family. They also become frustrated from a lack of resources in the community. Finally, there is little guidance in the literature that can provide direction for professionals in contact with developmentally disabled teenagers (Hammar and Barnard, 1966). This book is an effort to provide guidelines for planning individualized programs to assist the developmentally disabled adolescent to achieve maximum potential in the community. It is designed for the nurse and all members of a multidisciplinary team who individually or together must meet the daily challenges of the developmentally disabled adolescent.

## PREVALENCE OF DEVELOPMENTAL DISABILITIES

The prevalence of developmental disabilities is difficult to estimate because of ambiguous definitions and conditions, uncertainties in diagnosis, and difficulties in accurate case finding due to continued ignorance, social stigmas, and shame within society at large. Moreover, many of the disabilities overlap in their clinical manifestations as indicated in Figure 1. For example, many individuals with cerebral palsy may have a concurrent seizure disorder, while some persons who are intellectually impaired may have some emotional or behavioral problems (Seidel, 1976).

Mental retardation is one of the most prevalent developmental disabilities in the United States today, with 30 out of every 1,000 persons affected. It is estimated that approximately 120,000 children are born annually who are or will become retarded (Ehlers, 1973).

A recent summary of epidemiological surveys conducted in the United States concluded that the prevalence ratio was 0.3 percent of our total population for mental retardation. Included in this category was moderate, severe, and profound retardation (Tarjan, Wright, Eyman, and Kieran, 1973). Table 1 illustrates the various classifications and potentialities of the mentally retarded. Approximately 85%

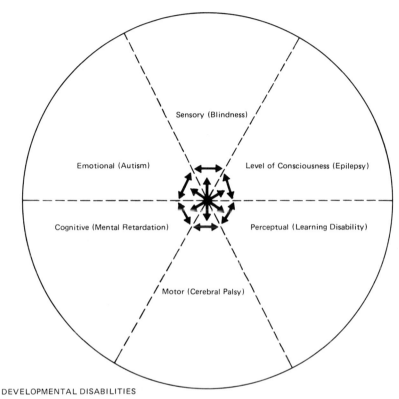

DEVELOPMENTAL DISABILITIES

Figure 1.    Overlapping of clinical manifestations of disabilities. From: Seidel, M. 1976. Career Development in the Health Professions: Nursing Care of Children with Mental Retardation and Other Developmental Disabilities. University of Washington School of Nursing and Child Development and Mental Retardation Center.

to 90% of these individuals have a mild handicap, live within the community, and lead a "normal" life, given early remediation and a therapeutic environment (Seidel, 1976). Tarjan and associates (1973) found that when mild retardation was added it affected the prevalence rate by reducing the numbers of affected adults found in the general population. Among the possible suggestions for such a discrepancy were: 1) changes in the definition of mental retardation, 2) different ways of identifying mildly retarded individuals, 3) confusion over what constitutes sociocultural retardation. Tarjan concluded that further epidemiological studies are required to explain the "disappearing retarded" in the adult age range.

Ten to 15% of the retarded population are more severely affected with major physical problems that may accompany or cause

Table 1.   Classifications and potentialities of the mentally retarded[a]

| Classi-fication | Estimated number | Percent | Potential behaviors |
|---|---|---|---|
| Mild | 5,340,000 | 89 | Educable, capable of working and living own life with support |
| Moderate | 360,000 | 6 | Trainable, can be taught to do useful tasks (sheltered workshops), may need some residential facilities and centers |
| Severe | 210,000 | 3.5 | Limited language and motor ability, may have physical disability, can learn certain basic self help skills, at home or in residential facility |
| Profound | 90,000 | 1.5 | Major physical impairment, require complete care, minimum self help skills |

[a] From Ehlers, W., Krishef, C., and Prothers, J. 1973. *An Introduction to Mental Retardation: A Programmed Text,* Charles E. Merrill Publishing Company, Columbus.

an intellectual impairment. More frequently than the general population, retarded persons have additional physical or emotional problems severe enough to constitute handicaps in themselves, as Figure 2 illustrates (Conroy and Derr, 1971).

In addition to the 6.4 million retarded individuals in our population, there are .75 million with cerebral palsy. Unknown numbers of these also suffer from epilepsy, sensory impairment, learning disabilities, and autism. Estimates have been made that there are 8.7 million children and adults who are considered developmentally disabled (Hobbs, 1975). The United States Office of Education has estimated that 7.9 million children from birth to age 19 are handicapped. Of these, 6.7 million are 6 to 19 years of age. Table 2 breaks down the estimated number of handicapped children identified by the Office of Education in 1976.

If the immediate families of the developmentally disabled individuals are also counted, the number grows to more than 20 million. Extended family members also increase the number of those affected by a developmental disability. The number of persons involved with

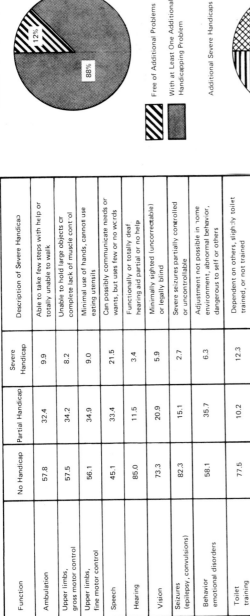

Additional Handicaps of Any Kind

88%

12%

◨ Free of Additional Problems

▨ With at Least One Additionally Handicapping Problem

Additional Severe Handicaps

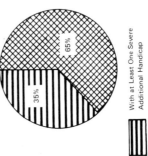

35%

65%

With at Least One Severe Additional Handicap

Free of Severe Additional Problems

| Function | No Handicap | Partial Handicap | Severe Handicap | Description of Severe Handicap |
|---|---|---|---|---|
| Ambulation | 57.8 | 32.4 | 9.9 | Able to take few steps with help or totally unable to walk |
| Upper limbs, gross motor control | 57.5 | 34.2 | 8.2 | Unable to hold large objects or complete lack of muscle control |
| Upper limbs, fine motor control | 56.1 | 34.9 | 9.0 | Minimal use of hands, cannot use eating utensils |
| Speech | 45.1 | 33.4 | 21.5 | Can possibly communicate needs or wants, but uses few or no words |
| Hearing | 85.0 | 11.5 | 3.4 | Functionally or totally deaf hearing aid partial or no help |
| Vision | 73.3 | 20.9 | 5.9 | Minimally sighted (uncorrectable) or legally blind |
| Seizures (epilepsy, convulsions) | 82.3 | 15.1 | 2.7 | Severe seizures partially controlled or uncontrollable |
| Behavior emotional disorders | 58.1 | 35.7 | 6.3 | Adjustment not possible in some environment, abnormal behavior, dangerous to self or others |
| Toilet training | 77.5 | 10.2 | 12.3 | Dependent on others, slightly toilet trained, or not trained |

Percentages may not add to 100 due to rounding.

Figure 2.  Prevalence of other handicaps in mentally retarded persons. Adapted from: Conroy, J. W., and Dorr, K. E. 1971. Survey and Analysis of the Habilitation and Rehabilitation Status of the Mentally Retarded with Associated Handicapping Conditions. Department of Health, Education, and Welfare, Washington, D.C.

Table 2.    Estimated number of handicapped children served and unserved by type of handicap[a]

| | 1975–76 served (projected) | 1975–76 Unserved | Total handicapped children served & unserved | Percent served | Percent unserved |
|---|---|---|---|---|---|
| Total: Age 6–19 | 3.86 | 2.84 | 6.7 | 58 | 42 |
| Total: Age 0–5 | .450 | .737 | 1.187 | 38 | 62 |
| Total: Age 0–19 | 4.31 | 3.577 | 7.887 | 55 | 45 |
| Speech impaired | 2.02 | .273 | 2.293 | 88 | 12 |
| Mentally retarded | 1.35 | .157 | 1.507 | 90 | 10 |
| Learning disabilities | .26 | 1.706 | 1.966 | 13 | 87 |
| Emotionally disturbed | .255 | 1.055 | 1.31 | 19 | 81 |
| Crippled and other health impaired | .255 | .073 | .328 | 78 | 22 |
| Deaf | .045 | .004 | .049 | 92 | 8 |
| Hard of hearing | .066 | .262 | .328 | 20 | 80 |
| Visually handicapped | .043 | .023 | .066 | 65 | 35 |
| Deaf-blind and other multi-handicapped | .016 | .024 | .040 | 40 | 60 |

[a] American Education, June 1976. Numbers expressed in millions.

the problem occupationally and professionally or in the interactions of daily life is impossible to calculate. Ultimately everyone is involved with the problem indirectly, in terms of helping to pay its social costs and in facing its not wholly predictable risks to every family (President's Committee on Mental Retardation (PCMR) 1976).

## THE ADOLESCENT PERIOD

The teenager with a developmental disability does not adjust easily to the bodily and psychological changes that accompany the onset of puberty. There are many developmental gaps which may prevent him from ever reaching the usual degree of maturation in some areas, but irregularities in development are not just the result of chance or individual difference (Morganstern, 1973). Interference with growth and development may be attributable to chromosomal defects, inborn errors of metabolism, genetic aberrations, and a whole host of other systemic disorders that affect the physical development of an individual child. Abnormal brain structure, maturation, or function can also impair the progress of normal development (Johnston and Magrab, 1976). The adolescent may see himself as a clumsy, awkward person who cannot compete with peers in gross motor activities like running or jumping, or in ordinary fine motor activities like cutting and wrapping (Morganstern, 1973).

On a psychosocial level, interference with development can be attributed to insufficient experience, indifference to the environment, environmental deprivation, or inability to shift thinking. The fear of ridicule may tend to segregate the disabled adolescent from his peers (Morganstern, 1973). Friends are apt to be themselves developmentally disabled or, possibly, younger children (Brier, 1975).

During this period, parents tend to feel overwhelmed by the manifestations of their child's physical and sexual growth. Some may urge their developmentally disabled child to grow up while at the same time attempting to prolong their son's or daughter's dependence. Parents may do this through actions based on conflicts in their own feelings concerning independence (Morganstern, 1973).

Ultimately, vocational, career, and life preparation should be vital aspects of individualized programs for the developmentally disabled adolescent. Training programs should assist them to become as competent and independent as possible. Such programs should enable the adolescent to take part in the regular community (Nirje, 1969).

## NORMALIZATION

Striving toward as normal a life as possible in the community has its roots in the concept of normalization. According to Braddock, the documentary origin of normalization principles in the English literature is attributed to Nirje (1969) and Wolfensberger (1972). Normalization refers to: "The concept of helping developmentally disabled persons to obtain an existence as close to the normal as possible, making available to them patterns and conditions of everyday life as close to the norms and patterns of society. Specifically [it refers] to use of the means that are culturally normative as possible to elicit and maintain behavior that is as culturally normative as possible" (National Association for Retarded Citizens, 1972).

Braddock contends that the normalization principle can be illustrated in three common service programs: living arrangements, educational alternatives, and employment alternatives (New Jersey Developmental Disabilities Council, 1975). The normative (or typical) living arrangement is depicted as a private individual's home. The normative educational placement is termed conventional education in a regular classroom. The typical mode of employment is labeled competitive, self-supporting employment. Contrasting these normative arrangements, at the abnormal ends of the service continuum, are congregate long term care institutions, homebound instruction, and no employment activity. Between these extremes lie many options, as illustrated in Figures 3, 4, and 5.

Braddock cautions that adhering to the normalization principle does not necessarily dictate that all living conditions and services should be identical for all disabled people in community settings. For some, the least prevalent but most disabled, there may not be a more normal alternative to long term care in a well programmed fifty bed residential facility. Competitive employment may be impossible, and education in a conventional setting may be ill-advised. Normalization is not a cure for disability but an orientation offering the "relative independence of the individual as the highest goal." Nirje (1970), aware of the possible misinterpretation of normalization as a magical cure, cautioned: "The application of the normalization principle will not make the subnormal normal but will make the life conditions of the mentally subnormal normal as far as possible, bearing in mind the degree of his/her handicap, his/her competence, and maturity, as well as the need for training activities and availability of services." Only relative independence is implied, and stressed by the words "as close to normal as possible." Normalization undoubtedly will guide many professionals concerned with the developmentally disabled in years to come. Of no less, if not greater, importance to the actual implementation of such ideals is the formulation of public policy that regulates what is clearly possible in developing programs for the developmentally disabled.

## PUBLIC POLICY FOR THE DEVELOPMENTALLY DISABLED

Programs and policies on behalf of the developmentally disabled have been slow to evolve. Total commitment to providing services across the board for all handicapped persons has come about only during the last 20 years. Such legislation has had its origins in the particular individual needs or pressures from specific disability groups, such as the blind or deaf. For example, the first bill relating to the handicapped to become national law had nothing to do with services for the handicapped, but provided authority to designate geographically a grant of land. The first part of the law pertained to lands reserved for a "seminary of learning" in the District of Florida, the second part to the location of the Deaf and Dumb Asylum of Kentucky (La Vor, 1976).

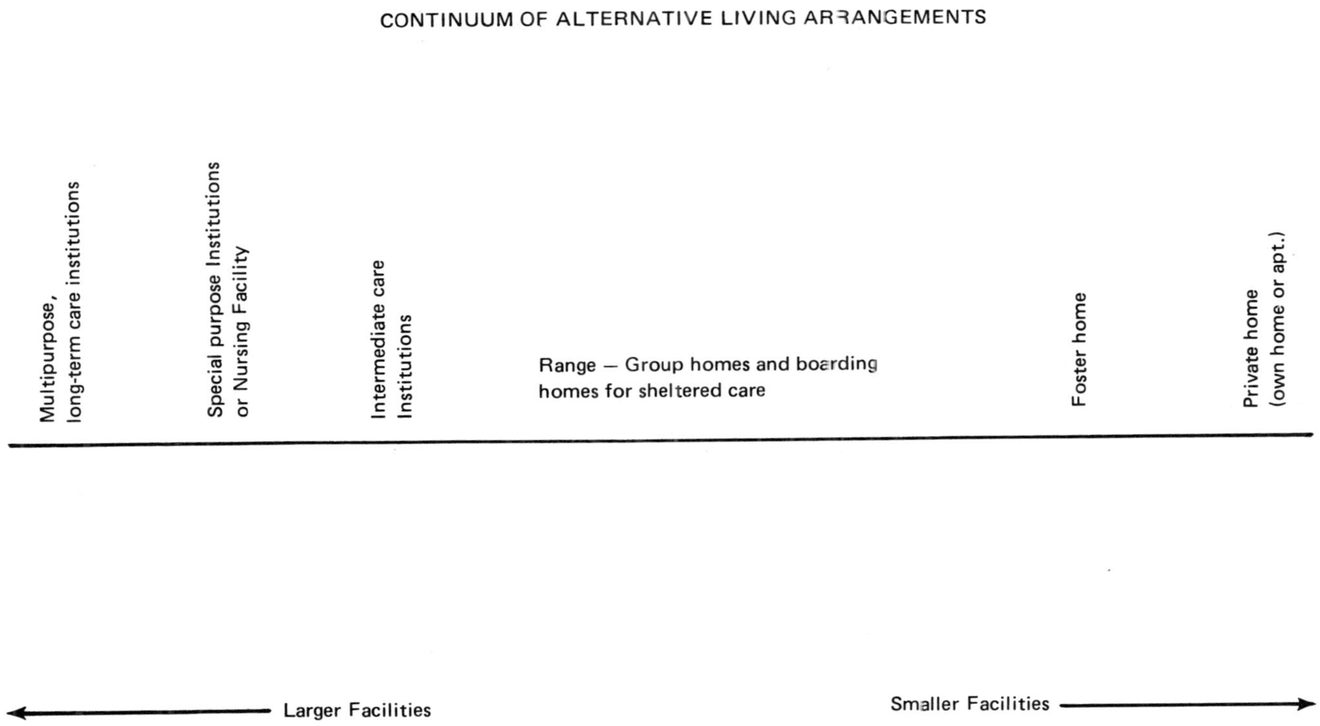

CONTINUUM OF ALTERNATIVE LIVING ARRANGEMENTS

Private home
(own home or apt.)

Foster home

Range — Group homes and boarding
homes for sheltered care

Intermediate care
Institutions

Special purpose Institutions
or Nursing Facility

Multipurpose,
long-term care institutions

Smaller Facilities

Larger Facilities

Figure 3.   Continuum of alternative living arrangements. From: The New Jersey Comprehensive Plan for the Developmentally Disabled, p. 5, 1975. New Jersey Developmental Disabilities Council, Trenton.

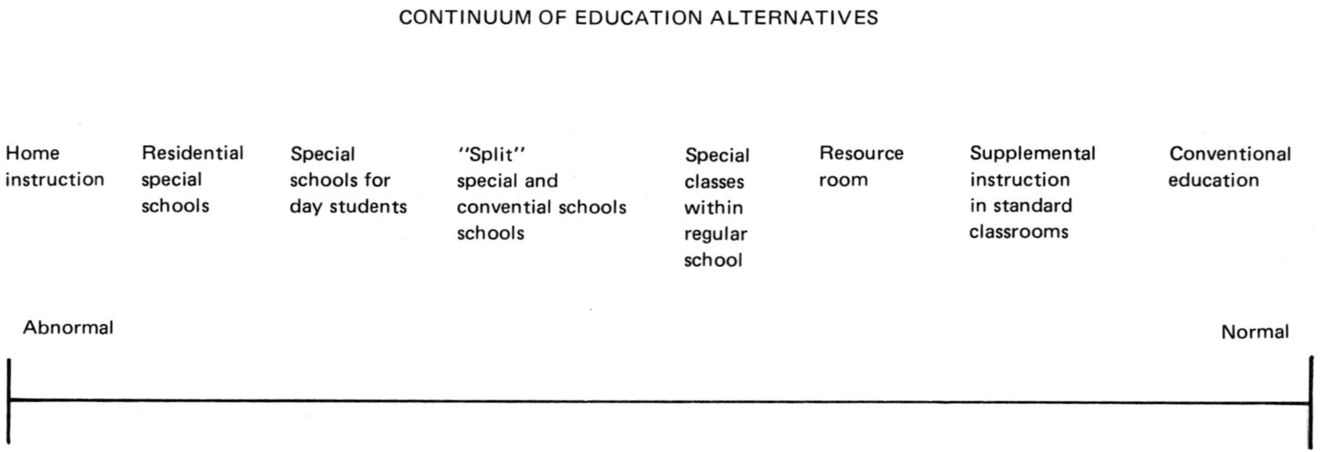

CONTINUUM OF EDUCATION ALTERNATIVES

Home instruction

Residential special schools

Special schools for day students

"Split" special and convential schools schools

Special classes within regular school

Resource room

Supplemental instruction in standard classrooms

Conventional education

Abnormal

Normal

Figure 4.   Continuum of education alternatives. From: The New Jersey Comprehensive Plan for the Developmentally Disabled, p. 6, 1975. New Jersey Developmental Disabilities Council, Trenton.

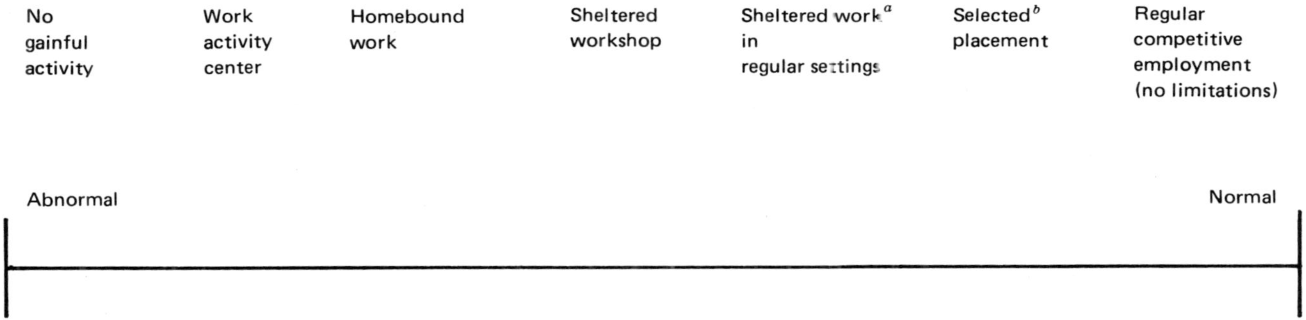

| No gainful activity | Work activity center | Homebound work | Sheltered workshop | Sheltered work[a] in regular settings | Selected[b] placement | Regular competitive employment (no limitations) |
|---|---|---|---|---|---|---|

Abnormal ├─────────────────────────────────────────────────────────────┤ Normal

Figure 5.  Continuum of employment alternatives. From: The New Jersey Comprehensive Plan for the Developmentally Disabled, p. 6, 1975. New Jersey Developmental Disabilities Council, Trenton.

[a] Sheltered work may mean work performed for less than the prevailing hourly rate, under special protective circumstances (such as different physical facilities), or at less than 50% productivity. [b] A regular job chosen from among a limited range of jobs suitable for the disabled person, including traineeships and apprenticeships.

In 1855 the first substantive law for the handicapped established a facility for the insane in the District of Columbia that came to be known as St. Elizabeth's. This facility was designed primarily for individuals who served with the Army or the Navy. The law also provided that residents of the District of Columbia, as well as non-residents under certain circumstances, could be admitted. It provided free services for natives, private care for non-native individuals who could pay, and care for those who became insane while imprisoned.

On February 16, 1857 "An Act to Incorporate the Columbia Institution of the Deaf and Dumb and the Blind" became the initial federal effort in education for the handicapped. This law authorized the federal government to grant tuition to an institution which provided education solely to the handicapped. This institution became known as Gallaudet College in 1954. The development of special legislation for these disabilities continued into the 1920s and 1930s.

The first significant federal act for the handicapped in the 20th century was the "Soldiers Rehabilitation Act," unanimously passed by Congress and signed by President Wilson (La Vor, 1976). It offered vocational rehabilitation services to veterans who became disabled as a result of World War I. Disabled civilians were not included. To include disabled civilians was considered neither practical nor the responsibility of the federal government. World War II provided new impetus for developing programs for the disabled. With the United States' involvement in the war, there occurred a manpower shortage at home. It was this shortage that made it possible for handicapped civilians to receive federal aid. In 1943 the Citizens Rehabilitation Program was expanded to provide services to the mentally retarded and mentally ill as well as the physically handicapped. In 1954 Congress added provisions establishing research, demonstration, and training programs to improve rehabilitation activities. In 1965 the program was extended to include services for a larger number of disabled persons. In 1967 the rehabilitation program was again extended to establish a national center for deaf-blind youths and adults, and to provide rehabilitation services to handicapped migrant workers and their families.

The Social Security Act was the next landmark. It became law in 1935. Although it was not originally designed for the disabled, it opened the door for provision of income and rehabilitation services for several categories of disabled individuals. When first passed the act established a trust fund to finance benefits for aged individuals who contributed to the fund during their working years. In subsequent years, the act was amended to include a disability insurance program for disabled workers who had contributed to the fund during their working years. Over the years, programs financed through general revenues were added to provide financial assistance and services to the needy, the blind, the aged, families with dependent children, and the permanently totally disabled. In 1965 several major health programs for low income aged, blind, and disabled individuals and families with dependent children were consolidated into a new program called Medicaid. At the same time, Medicare was created to provide medical services for the aged. In 1972 the various public assistance programs were consolidated under a new title establishing the supplementary security income program. Later, services from several titles of the act were reworked and consolidated under a new title, a federal-state program of social services for the aid to dependent children and supplementary security income program populations. The program required that its blind and disabled recipients under 65 be supplied with vocational rehabilitation services (La Vor, 1976).

Possibly the biggest assistance that the handicapped have ever received in terms of public acceptability and stimulus for further legislation, resulted from the fact that President Kennedy had a retarded sister and Vice-President Humphrey had a retarded grandchild. In 1961 as a result of the personal commitments of both men, the President appointed the "President's Panel on Mental Retardation" with a mandate to develop a national plan to combat mental retardation. Two years later legislation was passed that implemented several of the panel's recommendations.

In the years that followed, legislation was passed providing funds for states to develop state and community programs and to construct facilities to serve the mentally retarded. Funding was also made available for community mental health centers, research to provide demonstration centers for the education of the handicapped, and training of personnel to work with the handicapped through university affiliated programs.

Unquestionably, the parents' movement led to many reforms through the efforts of the Association for Retarded Citizens (ARC) and the National Association for Retarded Children (NARC). Their early goals revealed a commitment to dispel prevailing misconceptions about mental retardation with an intent to affect the public and professional establishments of the day. Emphasis was placed on research, professional training, and public information. Specific to the issue of needs, NARC aimed to have retarded people recognized, for purposes of economic needs, as "permanently and totally disabled." NARC also tried to have the mentally retarded accepted as "handicapped" for purposes of federal rehabilitation programs. NARC also strove to allow the mentally retarded to receive appropriate diagnosis and evaluation. State and local chapters of ARC were assisted in improving special education, residential care, and community support services (Cherington, 1974).

During the 1970s Congressional attention to the handicapped increased greatly. In 1972 the Congress extended the Vocational Rehabilitation Act of 1940. For the first time, state rehabilitation agencies were directed to give priority to "those individuals with the most severe handicaps." This act provided a greater role for the handicapped in determining their rehabilitation programs. It prohibited discrimination against any handicapped person in any program receiving federal assistance. The provisions of the 1972 Vocational Rehabilitation Act which passed both houses of Congress marked the first time in history that legislation for the handicapped had been vetoed by the President. The second version of the legislation, passed in 1973, was also vetoed. That veto was sustained by the Senate. Legislation agreeable to both branches was eventually enacted that retained the innovative features originally laid out in the 1972 Vocational Rehabilitation Act. In October, 1975 the "Developmentally Disabled Assistance and Bill of Rights Act" became law. It broadened the 1971 definition of developmental disabilities and the strategies for strengthening services and safeguarding individual rights. Public Law 93-380, the Education Amendments of 1974, required each state to establish a goal of providing full educational opportunity for all handicapped children, along with a comprehensive plan and time table for its achievement. The amendments increased funds available to states and broadened the rights of exceptional children and their parents.

On November 29, 1975, the President signed into law the Education for All Handicapped Children Act (PL 94-142). This Act committed the federal government to a substantial financial contribution toward the education of America's handicapped children, and it refined and strengthened those educational rights that had originally received attention in the earlier Public Law 93-380.

Despite the evolution of such public policies, legal safeguards, and appropriate advocacy programs that protect the rights of the developmentally disabled, further development is still needed. Most services for these individuals, both within institutions and in the community, suffer from a lack of adequately trained personnel. Parental finances are rapidly diminishing. Public assistance programs often place restrictions on the type and amount of treatment available. Insurance companies are reluctant to cover the chronically ill. Their comprehensive approach to service frequently includes a diagnosis but does not include well coordinated long term management and treatment (Seidel, 1976). Society has many more obstacles to overcome before the developmentally disabled have achieved the right and the means to develop to their fullest potential. Certainly with the magnitude of the physical and psychosocial problems facing the developmentally disabled, the nurse with a varied background in the physical and behavioral sciences must accept a growing responsibility in the treatment of this population.

## REFERENCES CITED

Braddock, D. 1976. Opening Closed Doors. The Deinstitutionalization of Disabled Individuals. The Council for Exceptional Children, Reston, Virginia.

Brier, N. M. 1975/76. Difficult hurdles for developmentally disabled teens. In: Rose F. Kennedy Center for Research in Mental Retardation and Human Development/Notes, Vol. 4, p. 2.

Cherington, C. 1974. Community life and individual needs. In: C. Cherington and G. Dybwad (eds.), New Neighbors: The Retarded Citizen in Quest of a Home, pp. 1-17. President's Committee on Mental Retardation, Washington, D.C.

Chinn, P. C., Drew, C. J., and Logan, D. R. 1975. Mental Retardation: A Life Cycle Approach, p. 179. C. V. Mosby, St. Louis.

Conroy, J. W., and Derr, K. E. 1971. Survey and Analysis of the Habilitation and Rehabilitation Status of the Mentally Retarded With Associated Handicapping Conditions. Department of Health, Education, and Welfare, Washington, D.C.

Ehlers, W., Krishef, C., and Prothers, J. 1973. An Introduction To Mental Retardation: A Programmed Text. Charles E. Merrill, Columbus.

Hammar, S. L., and Barnard, K. E. 1966. The mentally retarded adolescent: a review of the characteristics and problems of 44 non-institutionalized adolescent retardates. Pediatrics 38:845-857.

Johnston, R. B., and Magrab, P. R. 1976. Introduction to developmental disorders and the interdisciplinary process. In: R. B. Johnston and P. R. Magrab (eds.), Developmental Disorders: Assessment, Treatment, Education, pp. 3-12. University Park Press, Baltimore.

La Vor, M. L., 1976. Federal legislation for exceptional persons: a history. In: F. J. Weintraub, A. Abeson, J. Ballard, and M. L. La Vor (eds.), Public Policy and the Education of Exceptional Children, pp. 96-111. Council for Exceptional Children, Reston, Virginia.

Morganstern, M. 1973. The psychosexual development of the retarded. In: F. F. De La Cruz and G. D. La Veck (eds.), Human Sexuality and the Mentally Retarded, pp. 15-28. Brunner/Mazel, New York.

National Association for Retarded Citizens. 1972. ACFMR gives accreditation to 21 residential facilities. Ment. Retard. News 24:2.

New Jersey Developmental Disabilities Council. 1975. The New Jersey Comprehensive Plan for the Developmentally Disabled. Trenton, N.J.

Nirje, B. 1969. The normalization principle and its human management implications. In: Kugel and Wolfensberger, (eds.), Changing Patterns in Residential Services for the Mentally Retarded, pp. 181–195. President's Committee on Mental Retardation, Washington, D.C.

President's Committee on Mental Retardation. 1976. Mental Retardation: Century of Decision. U.S. Government Printing Office, Washington, D.C.

Seidel, M. S. 1976. Career Development in the Health Professions: Nursing Care of Children with Mental Retardation and Other Developmental Disabilities, p. 5. University of Washington School of Nursing and Child Development and Mental Retardation Center.

Stedman, D. J. 1971. Mental Retardation Programs in the Department of Health, Education, and Welfare. Report to the Secretary's Committee on Mental Retardation.

Tarjan, G., Wright, S. W., Eyman, R. K., and Keeran, C. V. 1973. Natural history of mental retardation: some aspects of epidemiology. Am. J. Ment. Defic. 77:369–379.

U.S. Department of Health, Education, and Welfare. Office of Human Development. Developmental Disabilities Program, The 1975 Amendments. Developmental Disabilities Office, Washington, D.C.

Wolfensburger, W. 1972. The Principle of Normalization in Human Services. University of York Press, Toronto.

# chapter two

# NURSES' RESPONSIBILITY IN ADOLESCENCE

Mary Lou de Leon Siantz, R.N., M.N.
and Jennie Downer Austin, R.N., B.S.

Early case finding of infants and children at risk for developmental disabilities has been a well established goal in nursing practice. Una Haynes (1969) has documented that the opportunity and responsibility for assisting with detection of deviation from normal patterns of growth and development are shared by all professional nurses who have any contact with children. Barnard and Erikson (1976) have also reported that nurses have primary responsibility in several major areas within the field of developmental disabilities. They have described these as prevention, serial observation, physical assessment, early programming, and management, as well as early case finding. As these children mature into adolescents, nursing practice should ensure continuation of care in order to facilitate and maintain maximal independence for the developmentally disabled adolescent within his own community. In general, nursing intervention with this group should include the following:

1. assessment
2. health maintenance
3. interdisciplinary approaches
4. goal directed treatment
5. inclusion of the developmentally disabled adolescent in the treatment formulation
6. case management
7. advocacy

## CONCEPTUAL FRAMEWORK

The concepts that provide guidelines for implementing these nursing responsibilities include a developmental approach, normalization, and mainstreaming.

According to the *developmental model,* development takes place in an orderly, sequential, and predictable manner. Every person has universal human needs that change according to age, capability, and development. These needs include shelter, health, physical development, personal and social growth (NARC, 1972). This model assumes that every person is capable of learning and that learning is indicated by a change in behavior that is not accounted for by maturation alone and that is augmented by reinforcement of that behavior. The aim is to facilitate and maintain as much independent functioning of the individual as possible (Cherington, 1974).

The theory of *normalization,* developed in Scandinavia, is a cluster of ideas, methods, and experiences that provides a pattern of life as close as possible to that which would be expected if the person did not have a handicap (Nirje, 1969). A related idea is *mainstreaming,* meaning the integration of handicapped and nonhandicapped persons in the same service structures whenever possible. Both ideas center on the provision of special assistance in the least restrictive setting and in the least stigmatizing manner possible. Both aim toward the maximum independence of the individual (Birch, 1974).

## ASSESSMENT

Assessment is the first step in the nursing process vital to initial development and periodic re-evaluation of individualized treatment plans for the developmentally disabled adolescent. It is during this phase that all relevant data are collected and documented for use in identifying needed subsequent evaluations, as well as in developing short term and long range treatment objectives for the individual. Assessment requires a comprehensive approach (Nirhira et al., 1975). It should include an intake, functional analysis, and home visit data.

### Intake

For the initial contact with the developmentally disabled adolescent and his parents or guardians, a thorough intake should begin the assessment process. Both the teenager and other persons in his environment are important sources of these historical data. The primary objective is to obtain a behavioral description that is representive of the total patient. The intake will offer clues about where to begin collecting more specific and objective baseline data. Where possible, birth history, physical, and developmental milestones should be reviewed. Due to time and memory, the parent/guardian, or the individual himself, may not have the information. Problems with speech, language, and hearing should be reviewed. Ability in fine and gross motor activities must be considered. Nutritional and dental status may be an area of concern for the growing adolescent. Educational, prevocational, and vocational factors should be reviewed. Social skills, including sexual behavior and independence in acts of daily living, should not be overlooked. The living environment is also a vital area requiring the nurse's review.

Appendix A at the end of the chapter illustrates an intake form used at the University Affiliated Program for Child Development, Georgetown University. While this is not a standarized form, it is meant for use as a guideline in gathering data that are helpful in identifying areas needing further evaluation by the nurse and other members of an interdisciplinary team that work with the developmentally disabled adolescent. In addition to the information identified by the intake form, it is important to note the individual's stage of adolescent development, since many developmentally disabled adolescents have the same physical attributes as their normal peers (Chinn, Clifford, and Logan, 1975). Age-appropriate behaviors can be determined by comparing the patient's behavior with a listing of developmental tasks such as that provided by Havighurst's *Developmental Tasks and Education* (1972). The individual nurse's judgment will help determine whether or not lack of a certain age-appropriate behavior is detrimental. An adolescent whose parents are unaware of but receptive to recreational programs, for example, has a better chance of optimal development than one whose parents refuse to allow his participation in such programs. Because case examples can help illustrate application of concepts, the following cases will be used to illustrate concepts used in this chapter.

*Case One*  Mr. R. is an obese 16-year-old, mildly mentally retarded male. He attends a special class in the local public school system. Mr. R. is functioning on a 5th to 6th grade level in school. He has glaucoma in his only eye. He is also diabetic with hypertension. He lives at home with a supportive and intact family that is motivated to facilitate his independence but that lacks awareness of areas in which to develop his independence. For example, his mother always administers his eye drops and insulin injections.

   *Case Two*   Miss S. is a 14-year-old, severely retarded female with cerebral palsy. She has a mild left hemiparesis. She attends a private school for the developmentally disabled. Miss S. functions on a 2–3 year level. Her verbal skills approximate those of a 5 year old. She lives at home with her mother who is devoted to her total care.

## Functional Analysis

A functional analysis evaluates many aspects of behavior which contribute to, and are a part of, total adaptation to the living environment. Functional behavior includes social adjustment, maturation, ability to learn self-care activities, and acts of daily living. Levels of measured intelligence and levels of adaptive behavior should both be included in the functional assessment. Intellectual functioning may be assessed by a psychologist using one or more of the standardized tests developed for that purpose. Adaptive behavior is defined as the effectiveness or degree to which the individual meets the standards of personal independence and social responsibility expected of his age and culture group (Grossman, 1973). While it is recognized that there is positive correlation between intelligence and adaptive behavior, demonstrations of variability in an individual indicate that separate measures are warranted (Chinn et al, 1975). This is especially true since it has become increasingly apparent that traditional tests of intelligence alone do not indicate how well an individual may function socially. Adaptive behavior ranges from mild to profound levels, as Table 1 illustrates. Since 1955, research has demonstrated that with behavioral and developmental techniques even higher levels of functioning can be achieved (Roos, 1975).

   A number of tests are currently available, such as the Vineland Social Maturity Scale, the AAMD (American Association on Mental Deficiency) Adaptive Behavior Scale, and the Balthazar Scales of Adaptive Behavior, which measure aspects of functional behavior contributing to total adaptation. Each of these tests provides information in many areas, including self-care activities, sensorimotor skills, language development, economic activity, number and time use, domestic activity, self-direction, vocational activity, responsibility, and socialization. Consideration is also given to opportunities available to the individual and others in the environment, as well as development of skills. A listing of appropriate responses present within the teenager's behavioral repertoire will give the nurse much

Table 1.  Developmental characteristics of mentally retarded persons

| Degrees of mental retardation | Pre-school age 0–5 maturation and development | School age 6–20 training and education | Adult 21 and over social and vocational adequacy |
| --- | --- | --- | --- |
| Mild | Can develop social and communication skills; minimal retardation in sensorimotor areas; often not distinguished from normal until later age. | Can learn academic skills up to approximately sixth grade level by late teens. Can be guided toward social conformity. "Educable." | Can usually achieve social and vocational skills adequate to minimum self support but may need guidance and assistance when under unusual social or economic stress. |
| Moderate | Can talk or learn to communicate; poor social awareness; fair motor development; profits from training in self-help; can be managed with moderate supervision. | Can profit from training in social and occupational skills; unlikely to progress beyond second grade level in academic subjects; may learn to travel alone in familiar places. | May achieve self-maintenance in unskilled or semi-skilled work under sheltered conditions; needs supervision and guidance when under mild social or economic stress. |
| Severe | Poor motor development; speech is minimal; generally unable to profit from training in self-help; little or no communication skills. | Can talk or learn to communicate; can be trained in elemental health habits; profits from systematic habit training. | May contribute partially to self-maintenance under complete supervision; can develop self-protection skills to a minimal useful level in controlled environment. |
| Profound | Gross retardation; minimal capacity for functioning in sensorimotor areas; needs nursing care. | Some motor development present; may respond to minimal or limited training in self-help. | Some motor and speech development; may achieve very limited self-care; needs nursing care. |

From *The Problem of Mental Retardation*, pp. 8–9. 1975. Office for Handicapped Individuals. President's Committee on Mental Retardation, Washington, D.C.

valuable information regarding the individual's assets (Loomis and Horsley, 1974).

The Vineland Social Maturity Scale provides an outline of detailed performance regarding which individuals show a progressive capacity for looking after themselves and for participating in those activities which lead toward ultimate independence as adults. The items are arranged in order of increasing average difficulty and age graded 0–25 years. Their content is arranged into areas of self-help, self-direction, locomotion, communication, and social relations.

Assessment is carried out by interviewing the parents and, if possible, observing the individual (Doll, 1965).

The AAMD Adaptive Behavior Scale is a behavior rating scale for mentally retarded, emotionally maladjusted, and developmentally disabled individuals. It can be used with other handicapped individuals as well. It is designed to provide objective descriptions and evaluations of an individual's adaptive behavior. This scale was developed with the idea that the manner in which an individual maintains his personal independence in daily living, or the ways in which he meets the social expectations of his environment are important pieces of information needed by those in charge of training and habilitation of retarded persons (Nirhira et al, 1975). The scale consists of two parts. Part one is organized along developmental lines. It is designed to evaluate an individual's skills and habits in areas considered important to the development of personal independence in daily living. Part two is designed to evaluate personality and behavior traits influencing the individual's ability to fulfill social expectations in his community or residential setting (Nirhira et al, 1975).

In the Balthazar Scales of Adaptive Behavior, section I, The Scales of Functional Independence, assesses the self help skills of the profoundly and severely mentally retarded. Specifically, the scales measure, rank, order, and classify a broad range of self-care behaviors which include eating, dressing, and toileting. Section II, The Scales of Social Adaptation, yields objective measures of coping behaviors. Specifically, section II comprises eight social scale categories: 1) unadaptive self directed behaviors, 2) unadaptive interpersonal behavior, 3) adaptive self-directed behavior, 4) adaptive interpersonal behavior, 5) verbal communication, 6) play activities, 7) response to instruction, and 8) check list items (Balthazar, 1973).

The Balthazar Scales of Adaptive Behavior can provide guidelines for the development of interdisciplinary treatment programs. It also affords a means to evaluate both quantitative and qualitative change. The scales are designed to determine the effectiveness of a given program or treatment technique. The test is administered through direct observation of the patient in his own environment. The patient is evaluated during typical daily activities, in familiar situations with familiar people. These conditions are particularly important for the more severely retarded who usually cannot adapt readily to unfamiliar settings or to formal test administrations that can be frustrating or threatening to them (Balthazar, 1973).

A note of caution is important concerning the use of both of these adaptive behavior scales, since they do have major limitations. They were developed primarily on institutional populations and do not adequately embrace the broad range of behaviors characteristic of mildly retarded individuals and others living in the community. Consequently, decisions must be based on a combination of pertinent test data, clinical observation, and utilization of all available sources of information regarding the individual's everyday behavior. Taking these factors into account, information from these scales is best utilized in an interdisciplinary setting in which all available services and disciplines are represented (Balthazar, 1973).

Finally, it must be stressed that in identifying individual program objectives, it is more important to gain information on the individual's performance on each set of behaviors rather than to establish a level of total adaptation. Since changes in adaptive behavior may occur either through treatment or through marked changes in the environment, reassessment at regular intervals is needed.

## Home Visit Data

The home visit is a traditional approach employed by many professional nurses. It remains a highly regarded method for assessment and practice. Ruth Freeman states that it permits the nurse to see the home and family situation in action. Such a visit can provide a more accurate appraisal of family relationships and competencies. It allows teaching in the actual situation without a need for the adolescent, parent, or guardian to make a transition from general instruction to their own facilities or equipment. The adolescent, family members, or guardian is less hesitant to raise questions than they might be in another situation, since they are not guests or patients in a strange environment. The nurse has the opportunity to observe how instructions are carried out as well as to assess how well the principles for a treatment program are understood. The adolescent gains confidence through direct personalized contact. Family members or guardians obtain support from the professional's presence (Freeman, 1966).

To achieve maximal effectiveness, home visits must be planned and thoughtfully executed. Observations should be selective and sensitive. The nurse needs to know what to look for in relation to the special needs of the particular disability and living environment. The home visit should include observation of the physical layout of the living environment and how it facilitates or inhibits the adolescent's continued progress. If adaptive equipment such as a wheelchair is used, an evaluation in the home of the physically handicapped person is needed. For example, if the wheelchair needs to be enlarged it is important to ascertain whether or not the wheelchair can fit through the doorway and bathrooms. Can the bathroom door be closed allowing privacy when the wheelchair is used? Can the adolescent close the door?

Since the adolescent must learn to function independently in his community, the nurse ought also to observe the community. Assessment should include: 1) means of transportation, 2) recreational facilities, 3) school and vocational resources, 4) proximity of banks, 5) postal facilities, and 6) health facilities.

The *Siantz/Austin Illustrated System Home Visit Guide* (the SAIS) is a form on which the nurse records observations of the adolescent's level of function in activities involving daily living skills. Although the guide is not standardized, it provides a convenient method of summarizing data typically identified during the course of a home visit. Through the use of the form, needs can be identified so that programs can be developed to increase the independence of the adolescent. It illustrates in a stylized manner four rooms with their furnishings. This is to allow for its use in any home environment of any size or structure. The four rooms portrayed are the bedroom, bathroom, kitchen, and an all purpose activity room. Below each illustration is a list of items typically found in that room. The nurse observes and rates the adolescent's independence in each task according to the scale presented. If a task is not directly observed by the nurse, but the parent reports to the nurse that the adolescent can perform the task, the nurse records R.B.P., that is, reported by parent, on the guide. Following the home visit, impressions and recommendations can be made. The use of a graphic representation helps to structure the home visit. It also is an effective means of communicating the need to modify the home environment to the interdisciplinary team and the parents. The interdisciplinary team will then be better able to visualize the home environment. The recommendations to the family and adolescent will be more effectively communicated through a concrete and pictorial manner. The guide is represented in its entirety with examples of how it can be adopted for use (Figures 1–6).

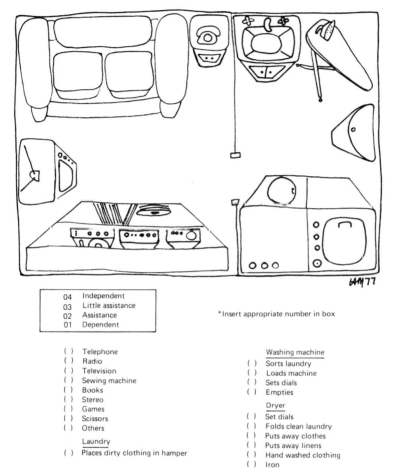

| 04 | Independent |
| 03 | Little assistance |
| 02 | Assistance |
| 01 | Dependent |

*Insert appropriate number in box

( )  Telephone
( )  Radio
( )  Television
( )  Sewing machine
( )  Books
( )  Stereo
( )  Games
( )  Scissors
( )  Others

Laundry

( )  Places dirty clothing in hamper

Washing machine

( )  Sorts laundry
( )  Loads machine
( )  Sets dials
( )  Empties

Dryer

( )  Set dials
( )  Folds clean laundry
( )  Puts away clothes
( )  Puts away linens
( )  Hand washed clothing
( )  Iron

Figure 1.  The Siantz/Austin Illustrated Home Visit Guide. The all purpose activity room.

## Alternatives to a Home Visit

If a home visit is not possible, there are two alternatives. One is to establish an acts of daily living apartment in the clinic or office for evaluations. The apartment can also double as a teaching area for the adolescent. The second alternative is to conduct an interview in order to collect data from the parent and adolescent. It is also possible in such an interview to observe interactions between family members.

Both alternatives have the disadvantage that the evaluator does not see the family in its natural environment.

### Three-Day Activity Record

Another tool for collecting information about the home is the 3-day activity record. The parents or the adolescent can fill out the form which describes how the adolescent spends his time over a 72-hour period. One of the days should be a Saturday or Sunday. The tool provides the nurse and the other professionals with an awareness of

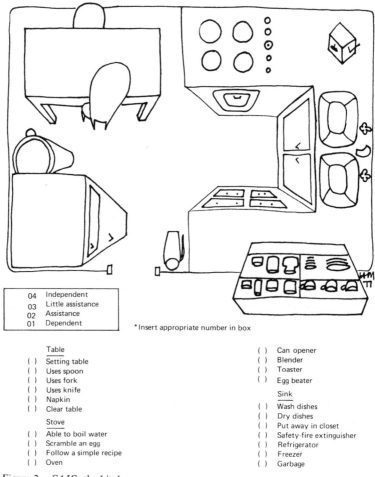

| 04 | Independent |
| 03 | Little assistance |
| 02 | Assistance |
| 01 | Dependent |

*Insert appropriate number in box

Table
( ) Setting table
( ) Uses spoon
( ) Uses fork
( ) Uses knife
( ) Napkin
( ) Clear table

Stove
( ) Able to boil water
( ) Scramble an egg
( ) Follow a simple recipe
( ) Oven

( ) Can opener
( ) Blender
( ) Toaster
( ) Egg beater

Sink
( ) Wash dishes
( ) Dry dishes
( ) Put away in closet
( ) Safety-fire extinguisher
( ) Refrigerator
( ) Freezer
( ) Garbage

Figure 2.   SAIS, the kitchen.

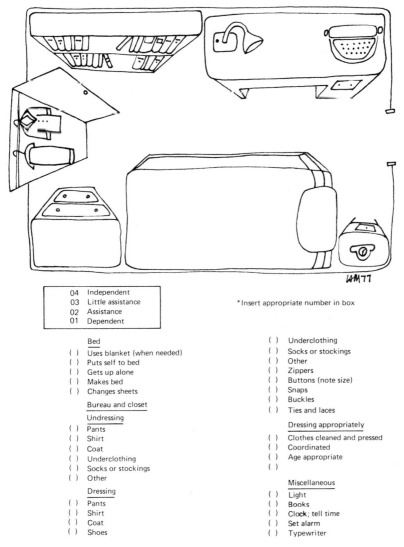

04  Independent
03  Little assistance
02  Assistance
01  Dependent

*Insert appropriate number in box

Bed
( )  Uses blanket (when needed)
( )  Puts self to bed
( )  Gets up alone
( )  Makes bed
( )  Changes sheets

Bureau and closet
Undressing
( )  Pants
( )  Shirt
( )  Coat
( )  Underclothing
( )  Socks or stockings
( )  Other

Dressing
( )  Pants
( )  Shirt
( )  Coat
( )  Shoes

( )  Underclothing
( )  Socks or stockings
( )  Other
( )  Zippers
( )  Buttons (note size)
( )  Snaps
( )  Buckles
( )  Ties and laces

Dressing appropriately
( )  Clothes cleaned and pressed
( )  Coordinated
( )  Age appropriate
( )

Miscellaneous
( )  Light
( )  Books
( )  Clock; tell time
( )  Set alarm
( )  Typewriter

Figure 3.   SAIS, the bedroom.

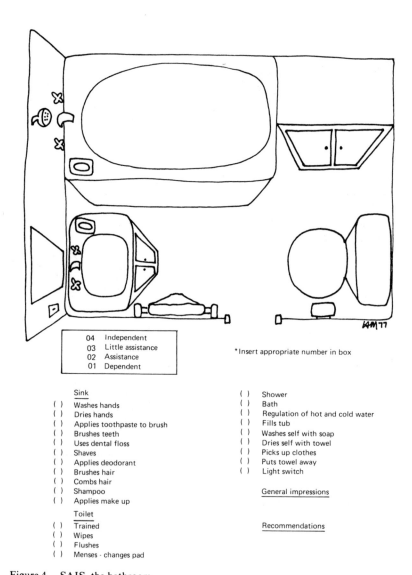

04  Independent
03  Little assistance
02  Assistance
01  Dependent

*Insert appropriate number in box

Sink
( )  Washes hands
( )  Dries hands
( )  Applies toothpaste to brush
( )  Brushes teeth
( )  Uses dental floss
( )  Shaves
( )  Applies deodorant
( )  Brushes hair
( )  Combs hair
( )  Shampoo
( )  Applies make up

Toilet
( )  Trained
( )  Wipes
( )  Flushes
( )  Menses - changes pad

( )  Shower
( )  Bath
( )  Regulation of hot and cold water
( )  Fills tub
( )  Washes self with soap
( )  Dries self with towel
( )  Picks up clothes
( )  Puts towel away
( )  Light switch

General impressions

Recommendations

Figure 4.   SAIS, the bathroom.

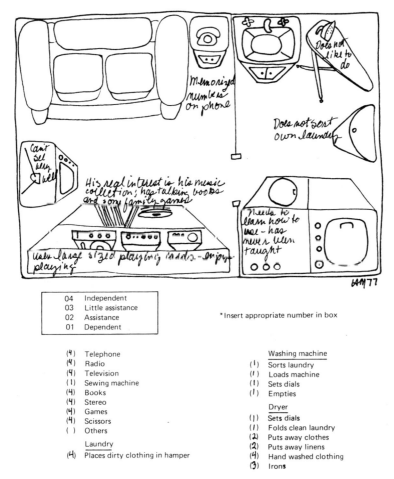

| 04 | Independent |
|----|-------------|
| 03 | Little assistance |
| 02 | Assistance |
| 01 | Dependent |

*Insert appropriate number in box

| ( 4 ) | Telephone |
|-------|-----------|
| ( 4 ) | Radio |
| ( 4 ) | Television |
| ( 1 ) | Sewing machine |
| ( 4 ) | Books |
| ( 4 ) | Stereo |
| ( 4 ) | Games |
| ( 4 ) | Scissors |
| ( ) | Others |

Laundry
| ( 4 ) | Places dirty clothing in hamper |

Washing machine
| ( 1 ) | Sorts laundry |
| ( 1 ) | Loads machine |
| ( 1 ) | Sets dials |
| ( 1 ) | Empties |

Dryer
| ( 1 ) | Sets dials |
| ( 1 ) | Folds clean laundry |
| ( 2 ) | Puts away clothes |
| ( 2 ) | Puts away linens |
| ( 4 ) | Hand washed clothing |
| ( 3 ) | Irons |

Figure 5.    Example 1—the all purpose activity room.

how the adolescent spends his free time and his structured time. One day of a 3-day activity record is presented for Mr. R. and Miss S.

One day of Mr. R.'s 3-Day Activity Record as recorded by himself Thursday AM:

  7–8:    I woke up and got dressed. Mom gave me my insulin and eye drops.
  8–9:    I ate breakfast and mother drove me to school.
  9–10:   In school.
  10–11:  In school.
  11–12:  I had swimming class.
  Noon:   I ate lunch alone.

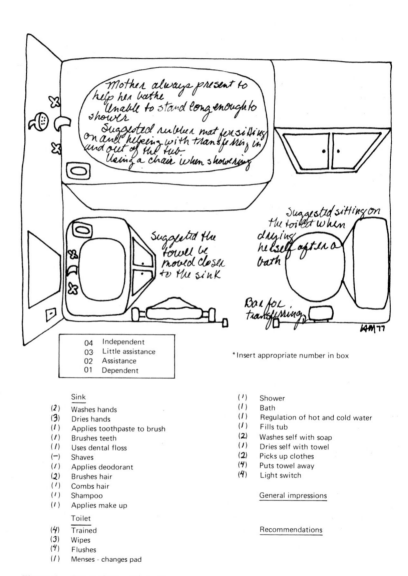

| | |
|---|---|
| 04 | Independent |
| 03 | Little assistance |
| 02 | Assistance |
| 01 | Dependent |

*Insert appropriate number in box

Sink

(2) Washes hands
(3) Dries hands
(1) Applies toothpaste to brush
(1) Brushes teeth
(1) Uses dental floss
(−) Shaves
(1) Applies deodorant
(2) Brushes hair
(1) Combs hair
(1) Shampoo
(1) Applies make up

Toilet

(4) Trained
(3) Wipes
(4) Flushes
(1) Menses - changes pad

(1) Shower
(1) Bath
(1) Regulation of hot and cold water
(1) Fills tub
(2) Washes self with soap
(1) Dries self with towel
(2) Picks up clothes
(4) Puts towel away
(4) Light switch

General impressions


Recommendations

Figure 6.    Example 2— the bathroom.

PM:
- 1–2:  I had a class in baking. We iced the cakes.
- 2–3:  We ate the cakes.
- 3–4:  Dad drove me home from school. We talked about our camping trip.
- 4–5:  I played cards in my room until my mother came home.
- 5–6:  Mom cooked dinner and I helped. I baked a cake for dinner.
- 6–7:  We had dinner. I talked to mom and dad about summer vacation. We want to go to California in the camper this summer.
- 8–9:
- 9–10:  I had cookies and a soda. I played records and played cards. I took a bath and brushed my teeth. Mom put my eye drops in and then I went to bed.
- 11–12:

AM:
- 12–1:  Asleep.
- 1–2:  Asleep
- 2–3:  Asleep.
- 3–4:  Asleep.
- 4–5:  Asleep.
- 5–6:  Asleep.
- 6–7:  Asleep.

From this 1-day record the nurse gains an awareness of Mr. R.'s daily activities. Some of her impressions are: 1) Mr. R. spends a great deal of time with his parents and rarely with peers his age, 2) he enjoys cooking and eating, and 3) his eye drops are administered by others.

One day of Miss S.'s 3-Day Activity Record as recorded by mother
Saturday AM:
- 7–8:  I'm awake. Miss S. is sleeping.
- 8–9:  I ate breakfast.
- 9–10:  Miss S. awoke. I gave her pancakes and she picked at them.
- 10–11:  I continued to sit with her until she finally finished. I sent her to her room to start getting dressed. I had put her clothes out on her bed.
- 11–12:  I had to remind her three times to dress and not to play. Finally I told her we would go out for lunch if she would get dressed. She got her underwear and socks on and I helped her with the rest. Her nightgown was wet from drooling.

PM:
- 1–2:  Lunch out. We went shopping for afternoon.
- 2–3:  Miss S. behaved well. She talked to many of the people in the
- 3–4:  stores.
- 4–5:  Returned home. Miss S. crying because she did not want to go home.
- 5–6:  Prepared dinner. I changed her shirt which was wet from drooling.
- 6–7:  Dinner served. Miss S. whining throughout dinner.

7–8:   Miss S. played alone in basement and then cleaned the fish tanks with me.

8–9:   Sent Miss S. to room to get undressed. She undressed herself. I gave Miss S. a bath and brushed her teeth. Then I told her to get in her pajamas but I had to help her.

9–10:  I kissed Miss S. goodnight, but she was up three more times.

10–11: Miss S. finally fell asleep.

11–12: Asleep.

AM:

12–1:  Asleep.

1–2:   Asleep.

2–3:   Called me for a glass of water.

3–4:   Asleep.

4–5:   Asleep.

5–6:   Asleep.

6–7:   Asleep.

In the case of Miss S. the nurse is aware that: 1) Miss S. spends all her free time with her mother, 2) she does not bathe independently, and 3) she is not provided with enough structured activities needed for independence in self-care.

## HEALTH MAINTENANCE

In the area of health maintenance the nurse should ensure either directly or by referral the periodic review of the following list cited by Braddock (1976):

1. health screening and health education
2. physical examination, including a thorough review of systems with neurologic, auditory, visual, and speech evaluation
3. dietary assessment with appropriate instructions to achieve optimal nutritional status
4. dental examinations and dental hygiene instruction as needed
5. drug counseling
6. family planning
7. genetic counseling
8. immunization
9. specialized equipment
10. speech and hearing therapy
11. physical and occupational therapy and physical education
12. optical prosthetics
13. motor prosthetics

Physical examinations carry a special significance for most teenagers who are usually aware of their developing bodies. Consequently, procedures should be described and explained and discussed in a concrete fashion utilizing diagrams and pictures along with simple rationale before they are performed. Ideally, the boy or girl should be permitted to state a preference about the sex of the examiner and the presence of chaperone. The follow-up of missed appointments should not give the impression of punitive surveillance but of positive participation in the adolescent's healthy status (Hammer, 1973).

## INTERDISCIPLINARY APPROACHES

Once sufficient assessment data have been collected to identify problem areas and goals, the nurse will be ready to share her impressions with an interdisciplinary team. The developmentally disabled adolescent, regardless of the diagnosis, rarely has a single problem that requires the service of only one professional. While there may be a few key people such as the parent, pediatrician, teacher, in the initial phases of identifying the disability, as the individual reaches adolescence, a wide range of professional support is still required for definitive diagnosis, problem identification, and treatment planning (Johnston and Magrab, 1976).

The physical therapist has the expertise to evaluate the present level of development and function of the individual in the area of posture and locomotion (Harryman, 1976). The occupational therapist's role involves specific areas of developmental deficiencies in the perceptual, adaptive, fine motor, and personal social skills which include ongoing social development and further establishment of self-help skills (Gorga, 1976). Traditionally, the speech pathologist has been trained to deal with the evaluation and management of speech disorders in children and adults. The audiologist evaluates and manages hearing disorders (Knobeloch, 1976). In addition to these professionals other specialists are needed to treat the adolescent. They include special education, vocational rehabilitation, dentistry, nutrition, psychology, medicine, social work, and law.

The ultimate goal in the delivery of service to the family with a developmentally disabled adolescent is a well coordinated interdisciplinary evaluation and habilitation plan. Whether the format is that of an ongoing interdisciplinary team, a monthly case conference staffing, or an informal referral system, the success of the overall evaluation treatment plan lies in the "shared communication" of the professionals involved (Johnston and Magrab, 1976). Hutchinson and Haynes (1969) have developed one model which they describe as transdisciplinary. Two conditions important to their concept are role extension and role release. This means that through the process of education and professional exchange there is a taking on of more complex activities within one's own disciplinary parameters (role extension) and giving up of some well established and traditional responsibilities to another discipline (role release).

An interdisciplinary team meeting provides an opportunity to consider the adolescent and his family from various points of view. The attitudes of every member of the professional staff have a marked effect on the adolescent's response to services. Individuals working with young people should be able to relate to them easily and from a nonjudgmental view point. Teenagers have stated that the professional discipline of the helping person does not matter, but that his personality and attitudes are highly important. Attention to emotional and social needs is no less important than attention to biological needs (Hoffman, 1975).

Serving the developmentally disabled is not easy. It provides a challenge to each professional involved to develop ways of working together collaboratively. Although every professional skill may not be essential in every case, it is from the selection and integration of all appropriate ones that effective planning and implementation proceed.

If the nurse is operating without benefit of an interdisciplinary team, she might look into the prospect of creating one or an approximation of one. For example, it may be within her responsibility to identify potential life skills programs and teen groups in the community and coordinate services with the adolescent, parent, or guardian. She can be alert to clues that the adolescent needs dental or nutritional counseling, or prevocational guidance, and refer the teenager to the appropriate discipline. An interdisciplinary approach provides the framework for comprehensive service (Barnard and Powell, 1974).

## FORMULATION OF TREATMENT GOALS

The combination of the nursing assessment and collaboration with an interdisciplinary team provides a definition of the nursing problems which, in turn, should lead to the establishment of treatment goals (Brill, 1973). Sound goals will give direction to nursing intervention. In beginning to formulate treatment goals, the nurse needs to recognize the individual's readiness to learn the task. The adolescent should be physically, mentally, and emotionally ready for the selected goal, and parents or guardians should be ready to support the goals as well. Determining the adolescent's readiness to learn a task is a major step in self help training. Limitations that affect training should be clearly identified (Kluss, 1976).

In our examples, Mr. R.'s glaucoma and Miss S.'s mild left hemiparesis were limitations needing consideration in planning goals. Intellectual ability will also influence how a training program is to be conducted. With Mr. R., who functioned on a sixth grade level, discussion was an important part of implementing treatment goals. With Miss S., functioning on a two to three year level, a more structured approach with simple demonstration and reinforcement was more appropriate.

Three of the many nursing problems identified with Mr. R. were: 1) lack of exercise, 2) no opportunity available to administer own eye drops, 3) lack of age-appropriate leisure activities. The goals established were daily exercise, instruction on administration of eye drops, and peer contact at home during free time. Mr. R. was expected to exercise daily in order to decrease his weight, improve his strength and coordination, and increase his endurance. Peer contact during leisure periods was important to develop appropriate social skills with his peer group. In order to teach him to administer his eye drops the following plan was used:

1. home visit to review Mr. R's understanding of his glaucoma and need for eye drops
2. discuss need for him to assume responsibility of administering eye drops with his parents
3. demonstrate use of eye dropper
4. return demonstration by Mr. R.
5. supervision until task is accomplished successfully
6. weekly chart kept by Mr. R. to show frequency of self administered eye drops
7. weekly sessions with nurse to evaluate progress in learning task

Mr. R. particularly enjoyed the degree of independence he felt in administering his own eye drops and verbalized this to the nurse. He stated that he had had questions regarding his vision in the past, but had been afraid to ask his parents or the physician. His parents began to realize that their son was capable of learning to take care of himself and began to ask how they might provide more opportunities for him to do so.

For Miss S., two of the several nursing problems identified were drooling and inability to bathe independently. The goals were to control drooling and to bathe alone. Miss S. was expected to decrease drooling since by so doing she would increase her acceptability in social and school situations. Drooling drew negative attention and created an unhygienic situation for her. Bathing was important to her health and cleanliness. The first step in the bathing process was to learn how to wash her face. The following program was formulated:

1. Miss S. brings hands to face with wet wash cloth
2. wipes face with water
3. picks up soap and applies soap to wash cloth
4. puts soap down
5. washes face with soapy wash cloth
6. rinses face
7. dries face

With Miss S., videotaping in the clinic setting with instant play back for her to observe correct and incorrect motions proved to be an excellent means of teaching and reinforcement. Ignoring Miss S. when incorrect behavior occurred was also very effective, since she enjoyed interacting with the nurse. A lack of opportunity for independent bathing had also contributed to Miss S.'s inability to bathe. The goal took three months to accomplish with weekly clinic visits. Weekly home visits for follow-up and parent training were also involved. During this period, progress was slow and at times barely noticeable, even to the point of occasional regression. The team support from others working with Miss S. proved to be a strong source of encouragement.

The techniques used in teaching the developmentally disabled adolescent will vary with the individual. Many techniques are available, such as behavior modification which Dr. Katz discusses in chapter 4, and which was useful with Miss S. Tasks can also be broken down into their simplest steps. Instruction, demonstrations, and practice sessions are important; videotape pictures and slides can be used for teaching. In general, treatment goals should become a routine part of the teenager's daily activities. Any equipment used should be kept as simple as possible. With Mr. R., only a bottle and eye dropper were used. With Miss S. a wash cloth, sink, towel, soap, and dish were used. A rubber mat was needed in the tub for safety and to improve stability for transfer.

## INCLUSION OF THE DEVELOPMENTALLY DISABLED ADOLESCENT IN THE TREATMENT FORMULATION

Goal setting is most effective when it is a shared process; when the patient has a major voice in deciding what needs to be achieved and how it is to be done. Motivation and independence are strengthened by this involvement. With Mr. R., the nurse asked him if he would like to learn how to administer his own eye drops. He was also asked if he would like to come to the clinic alone for the program. He became very excited with the prospect of doing this himself. Miss S. was told in very simple terms that we would like to teach her how to wash her face so that she could be a "big girl" like "Cher" whom she idolized.

Nurses and other health care professionals must avoid reinforcing passivity, dependency, and social isolation among the developmentally disabled adolescent. These factors are the most damaging to the possibilities of social rehabilitation. By rewarding the differences, incapacities, and dependency of these individuals, professionals fail to recognize that they reinforce the notion of doing something *for* the individual instead of *with* him (Katz, 1970). All too often health professionals choose to focus on the problematic or sick behavior of an individual. By doing so, they fail to fully utilize the behavioral assets which the person brings with him. Depending on the degree of discrepancy between the clinic environment and the teenager's home environment, those behavioral assets might be ignored. Inappropriate behaviors can often be easier to cite while strengths are overlooked or taken for granted. If nurses accept responsibility for facilitating and maintaining maximal independence for adolescents, it is vital that nurses involve the adolescent in planning the treatment program to the extent he is able to do so.

## CASE MANAGEMENT

Case managers can play an important role in involving the adolescent in his treatment program, since they will have the most consistent contact with him and are the key professionals involved with implementation of treatment goals (Johnston and Magrab, 1976). In selecting a case manager, the kind of ongoing care that will be needed must be carefully considered. Because of their varied background in the physical and behavioral sciences, nurses are well prepared to assume case management of developmentally disabled adolescents (Seidel, 1976).

Case managers will often have the responsibility of providing information, referral, and follow-up treatment as well as serving as an advocate when there are barriers in the service delivery system (Moore, 1976). Success or failure to reach short term goals can periodically be evaluated with long term goals in mind. Anticipatory guidance can be provided to the adolescent, parent, or guardian.

In particular, nurses can help manage common problems in acts of daily living, health, self-care, and adaptation to a new living environment. Management of such problems is particularly important to the developmentally disabled adolescent since independence in these areas is considered as valuable for them as it is for all persons in our society. The developmentally disabled adolescent who is accomplished in self-help skills is not only less dependent on others but also more acceptable to them and therefore, he does not need to feel as different as he once did. Examples of two adolescents working with a nurse to gain independence in activities of daily living are shown in Figures 7 and 8.

## ADVOCACY

Advocacy is not a new concept. Broadly defined, it refers to any activity which involves a person acting on his own behalf, or on the behalf of others, to secure responses to perceived needs. Early advocates might have been family members or the extended family of nomadic tribes. Although the concept of advocacy itself is simple, it becomes complex when one considers the wide range of functions which might be delegated to advocacy programs. Advocates can act as friends, parents, legal guardians of persons or estates, and case managers. These responsibilities have been delegated to parents, relatives, public officials, and agency personnel (Boggs, 1976).

The ability to serve as one's own advocate is one of the signs of maturity, and it is an essential component of social competence. The development of self-advocacy skills is one of the objectives of education for all. By instinct, by social custom, and by law, the family is a mutual advocacy system, whose members spontaneously act as advocates for one another as needed. Spouses serve as advocates for each other and parents are advocates for minor children.

If an individual is developmentally disabled, self-advocacy skills are likely to need supplementation for two reasons. First, there is likely to be an impairment of the individual's own ability to advocate for himself, which may be due to impairment of adaptive behavior,

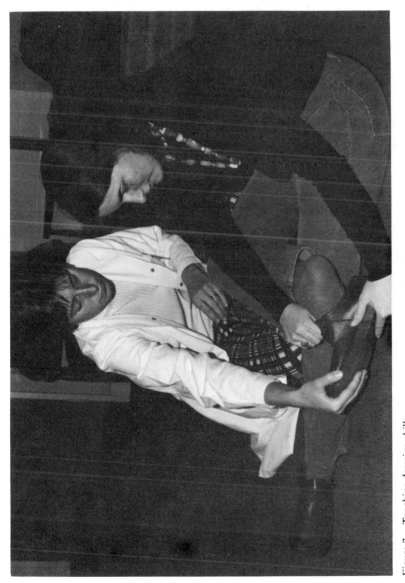

Figure 7.    Teaching dressing skills.

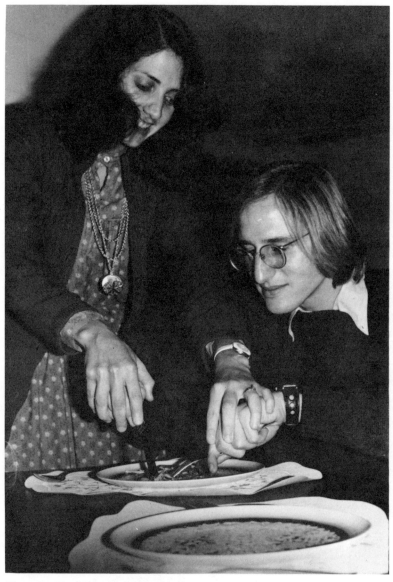

Figure 8.   Teaching use of knife and fork.

atypical experiences during the developmental period, or some handicap which may not impair him intellectually, but which may make it difficult for him to assert himself. Second, the array of services needed by the developmentally disabled is very complex, if incomplete, and there is often more available to the developmentally disabled and his family than they are aware of. For example, Mr. R.'s parents were unaware of recreational opportunities available to their son.

Advocacy should not inhibit any appropriate level of self-determination. Rather it should enhance such opportunities. Nevertheless, individuals with developmental disabilities, particularly those with the most serious forms of adaptive impairment, will need special advocacy (Boggs, 1976). In chapter 12, Bertram R. Cottine discusses specific ways that the nurse can act as an advocate for the disabled adolescent.

Most professions have codes of ethics which articulate the normative behavior expected of their members. However, the codes are usually limited in their articulation of the advocacy relationship between the professional and the child or adolescent. Weintraub (1976) in *Public Policy and the Education of Exceptional Children* outlined several principles for discussion by individual professionals concerned with the developmentally disabled population. He warned that these principles should be cautiously applied in practical situations. According to Weintraub (1976) these principles include:

1. reporting to the system the needs of the child
2. demanding from the system the appropriate resources to meet the needs of the child
3. challenging required participation in any activities that are inappropriate to the needs of the child
4. informing children and parents, guardians, and surrogates of their rights and any proposed or practiced violations of those rights
5. cooperating fully in administrative or judicial proceedings regarding a child
6. refraining from participating in any activities that require professional skills that you do not possess
7. seeking appropriate administrative or judicial action against other professionals who violate the rights of children
8. participating in political activities that will improve conditions necessary to better meet the needs of the child
9. seeking through contract negotiation appropriate conditions to

better meet the needs of the child and to engage in activities to prevent such contracts from abridging the rights of the child

10. expressing publicly views on matters affecting children
11. honoring requirements of confidentiality regarding the child and his or her family
12. working with other professionals to create an appropriate educational program in the least restrictive environment for all exceptional children

## REFERENCES CITED

Balthazar, E. E. 1971a. Balthazar Scales of Adaptive Behavior for the Profoundly and Severely Mentally Retarded: Section One, Part One: Handbook for the Professional Supervisor. Research Press, Champaign, Ill.

Balthazar, E. E. 1971b. Balthazar Scales for the Profoundly and Severely Mentally Retarded: Section One, Part Two: Handbook for the Rater Technician. Research Press, Champaign, Ill.

Balthazar, E. E. 1971c. Balthazar Scales for the Profoundly and Severely Mentally Retarded: Section One, Part Three: Program Scoring Form. Research Press, Champaign, Ill.

Balthazar, E. E. 1973. Balthazar Scales of Adaptive Behavior II: Scales of Social Adaptation. Consulting Psychologist Press, Palo Alto, Cal.

Barnard, K. E. and Erickson, M. L. 1976. Teaching Children with Developmental Problems: A Family Care Approach. Second ed. C. V. Mosby, St. Louis.

Bergman, Alan. A Guide to Establishing an Activity Center for Mentally Retarded Persons.

Birch, J. W. 1974. Mainstreaming: Educable Mentally Retarded Children in Regular Classes. Council for Exceptional Children, Reston, Virginia.

Boggs, E. 1976. Advocacy and Protective Services: Where Are We Coming From? In: C. J. Bensberg and C. Rude (eds.), Advocacy Systems for the Developmentally Disabled. Proceedings of the National Conference on Establishing Statewide Advocacy Systems as Required by the Developmentally Disabled Assistance and Bill of Rights Act. March 31–April 2, 1976. Dallas, Tex.

Braddock, D. 1976. Opening Closed Doors: The Deinstitutionalization of Disabled Individuals. The Council for Exceptional Children, Reston, Va.

Brill, N. I. 1973. Working with People The Helping Process. J. B. Lippincott, Philadelphia.

Cherington, C. 1974. Community Life and Individual Needs. In: Cherington and Gunnevar Dybwad (eds.), New Neighbors, pp. 1–17. President's Committee on Mental Retardation, DHEW Publication (OHD)74-21004.

Chinn, P. C., Drew, C. J., Logan, D. R. 1975. Mental Retardation: A Life Cycle Approach. C. V. Mosby, St. Louis.

Doll, E. A. 1974. Vineland Social Maturity Scale. Educational Test Bureau, Minneapolis.

Freeman, R. B. 1966. Public Health Nursing Practice. Third ed. W. B. Saunders, Philadelphia.

Gorga, D. I. 1976. Occupational therapy. In: R. B. Johnston and P. R. Magrab (eds.), Developmental Disorders: Assessment Treatment, Education. University Park Press, Baltimore.

Grossman, H. J. 1973. Manual on Terminology and Classification in Mental Retardation. American Association on Mental Deficiency, Washington, D.C.

Hammer, S. L. 1973. The approach to the adolescent patient. Pediatric Clinics of North America, Symposium on Adolescent Medicine. 20:779–788.

Harryman, S. E. 1976. Physical therapy. In: R. B. Johnston and P. R. Magrab (eds.), Developmental Disorders Assessment, Treatment Education, pp. 167–189. University Park Press, Baltimore.

Havighurst, R. J. 1972. Developmental Tasks and Education. Dean McKay, New York.

Haynes, U. 1969a. A Developmental Approach to Casefinding. Public Health Service, Publication 2017.

Haynes, U. 1969b. The First Three Years: Program for Atypical Infants. Report of a Nationally Organized Collaboration Project to Improve Services for Atypical Infants and Their Families, United Cerebral Palsy Association Inc., New York.

Hoffman, A. D. 1974. Health Care of inner-city Adolescents. Clin. Pediatr. 13:570–573.

Johnston, R. B., and Magrab, P. R. 1976. Developmental Disorders: Assessment, Treatment, Education. University Park Press, Baltimore.

Katz, A. H. 1970. Marginal man and the Status of the Handicapped in Our Society. In: The Second Milestone, pp. 38–50. United Cerebral Palsy Association, Inc., New York.

Kluss, K. 1976. Training the mentally retarded child in self held skills. In: P. A. Brandt, P. L. Chinn, M. E. Smith (eds.), Current Practice in Pediatric Nursing, pp. 57–175. C. V. Mosby, St. Louis.

Knobeloch, C. 1976. Speech and language. In: R. B. Johnston and P. R. Magrab (eds.), Developmental Disorders: Assessment, Treatment, Education. University Park Press, Baltimore.

Loomis, M. E., and Horsley, J. A. 1974. Interpersonal Change: A Behavioral Approach to Nursing Practice. McGraw-Hill, New York.

Moore, M. 1976. A demonstration of three advocacy models for persons with developmental disabilities. In: G. J. Bensberg and C. Rude (eds.), Advocacy Systems for the Developmentally Disabled, pp. 113–121. Proceedings of the National Conference on Establishing Statewide Advocacy Systems as Required by the Developmentally Disabled Assistance and Bill of Rights Act. March 31–April 2, 1976. Dallas, Tex.

National Association for Retarded Children, 1972. Residential Programming for Mentally Retarded Persons, A Developmental Model for Residential Services. National Association for Retarded Children, Arlington, Tex.

Nirhira, K., Foster, R., Shellhaas, M., and Leland, H. 1975. Adaptive Behavior Scale. American Association on Mental Deficiency, Washington, D.C.

Nirje, B. 1969. The normalization principle and its human management implications. In: R. B. Kugel and W. Wolfensberger (eds.), Changing Patterns In Residential Services For the Mentally Retarded, pp. 181–195. President's Committee on Mental Retardation, Washington, D.C.

Roos, P. 1975. The Severely and Profoundly Retarded: Past and Future. Paper presented at conference on Education of Severely and Profoundly Retarded Students, March 31–April 2, 1975. New Orleans.

Seidel, M. A. 1976. Career Development in the Health Professions: Nursing Care of Children With Mental Retardation and Other Developmental Disabilities. University of Washington School of Nursing and Child Development and Mental Retardation Center. Seattle.

Weintraub, F. J., and McCaffrey, M. A. 1976. Professional rights and responsibilities. In: F. J. Weintraub, A. Abeson, J. Ballard and M. L. La Vor (eds.), Public Policy and the Education of Exceptional Children, pp. 333–343. The Council for Exceptional Children, Reston, Va.

Appendix A
UNIVERSITY AFFILIATED PROGRAM FOR
CHILD DEVELOPMENT
Georgetown University
Interdisciplinary Intake
Interview Outline


Case history forms generally contain questions in the categories listed below. In your report please group information using the seven major headings and end with a separate section of recommendations. Please note that some questions apply only to certain age groups. Also note that some questions do not need to be asked in certain cases. Please begin by noting the name(s) of informant(s), the chief concern of the parent(s) and the chief concern of the referral source.


Check positive
indications for:

BIRTH HISTORY
_____ a. Pregnancy: length, condition of mother, unusual factors, medications, special procedures performed including x-ray, amniocentesis, etc.
_____ b. Birth conditions: term or premature, duration of labor, weight, unusual circumstances.
_____ c. Conditions following birth: jaundice, respiratory distress, need for oxygen, feeding problems.

PHYSICAL AND DEVELOPMENTAL DATA
_____ a. Health history: note any accidents, high fevers, other illnesses, hospitalizations.
_____ b. Present health: note habits of eating and sleeping, energy and activity levels, medications taken, specialists routinely consulted.
_____ c. Developmental history: note when first held head up, crawled, sat alone, walked, babbled, used first words, used first two-word sentences.
_____ d. Note family history of mental retardation, seizure disorders, delayed language, cerebral palsy, etc.
_____ e. Note name and address of physicians on information request and release forms.

SPEECH, LANGUAGE AND HEARING
_____ a. Hearing: are parents concerned about hearing? does child respond to telephone, listen to TV, respond when called from a distance? is there a history of upper respiratory infection or earaches or infection? how often?

Appendix A   (*continued*)

—————————    b.  Speech and language: are parents concerned about speech and/or language?

—————————    c.  Speech production: how easy is it to understand him?

—————————    d.  Language comprehension: does child understand what is said to him? does he follow instructions—with or without gestures? can he answer questions appropriately? does he relate verbally what happened? does he understand a story or TV plot?

—————————    e.  Language expression: number of words in his vocabulary; does child use appropriate labels or does he tend to use "thing" or "stuff" in place of nouns? what is length of utterances? are words in proper order? does child use pronouns, plurals, proper verb tenses? can he express his ideas in logical sequence?

—————————    f.  Voice quality: nasal, hoarse or breathy?

—————————    g.  Rate and rhythm: too fast, too slow, "stuttering"?

—————————    h.  Are the child's speech and language skills as good as those of other children his age?

—————————    i.  If problems exist, is the child aware of his own difficulties?

—————————    j.  What languages are spoken in the home?

### MOTOR SKILLS

—————————    a.  Are parents concerned about child's gross and fine motor skills?

—————————    b.  Does child show any clumsiness, awkwardness, or lack of coordination and balance?

—————————    c.  Does child have the ability to plan and execute skilled motor acts (ride tricycle or bicycle, dress and undress, etc.)?

—————————    d.  Does child have any abnormal types of movements, abnormal muscle tone, or orthopedic problems?

—————————    e.  Can child perform fine motor tasks such as using a pencil with proper grasp, cutting with scissors, putting toys together, etc.?

—————————    f.  Does child show a preference for gross motor activity (climbing, etc.?)

—————————    g.  Does he enjoy quiet activities such as blocks and puzzles?

### NUTRITION

—————————    a.  Are parents concerned about their child's eating habits or state of nutrition?

—————————    b.  Does child have any unusual food habits such as pica, eating snacks only, eating no vegetables, etc?

Appendix A   (*continued*)

—————————— c.  Does the child have any difficulty in sucking, swallowing, chewing; does he drool frequently?
—————————— d.  Is child excessively over- or underweight? What is child's current weight and height?
—————————— e.  Is child's skin very pale or rough and dry or puffy?
—————————— f.  Has the child ever been diagnosed as being anemic?

PATIENT/FAMILY SOCIAL FUNCTIONING
—————————— a.  Are parents concerned about the child's emotional state especially in regard to: anxieties, fears, dependency, aggression, withdrawal, reliability, enuresis, mood swings?
—————————— b.  Are parents concerned about familial interactions, relationships with peers, other outside social groups?
—————————— c.  Do parents perceive problems in the areas of patient's method of handling tasks and stresses—successes and failures both in the past as well as present?
—————————— d.  Do parents recognize strengths as well as weaknesses in patient and family?
—————————— e.  Are parents concerned about discipline?
—————————— f.  Is there parental agreement about child-rearing methods?
—————————— g.  Is there motivation and potential for patient/family change?
—————————— h.  Is there capacity to become involved in the process of change?

EDUCATIONAL FACTORS
—————————— a.  Are parents concerned about child's school experience?
—————————— b.  What is the chronology of child's school experience (nursery, kindergarten, grade school, etc.)? has child skipped or repeated any grades, moved, changed teachers in mid-year or received special help or special placement?
—————————— c.  Has any special testing been performed? when? where? by whom? (Note name and address of professional conducting evaluation and obtain parents' permission to request information on the appropriate form.)
—————————— d.  Do parents perceive any school problems? are they academic or behavioral in nature? has teacher contacted parents about problems? (Note on request for information form permission to talk to teacher and note name and address of teacher and school on confidential face sheet.)

Appendix A   (*continued*)

_____ e.  What are parents' perceptions of problems and
                            attitudes toward teacher and school?
_____ f.  Does the child have any complaints about going to
                            school, his teacher or classmates?

RECOMMENDATIONS:

# chapter three
# PHYSICAL DEVELOPMENT

Richard Jones, M.D.

Human biological development is marked by two periods of rapid growth: first is that of intrauterine differentiation and growth which continues unabated through delivery and the first 2 years of life. Thereafter follows a relatively constant but less active growth period during the childhood years. The second significant growth period occurs during adolescence. It is responsible in most cases for the final 20–25% of linear growth and almost 50% of ideal body weight (Barnes, 1975). Inextricably linked to this physical growth are the physical and psychological changes that so characteristically mark the differences between child and adult. Care of the adolescent must be based on a fundamentally sound knowledge of the normal physiological, anatomical, and psychosocial developmental changes that occur during the growth from childhood to adolescence. With a thorough understanding of the adolescent's growth pattern health care professionals can begin to comprehend the alterations that occur when physical and/or developmental abnormalities either alter, retard, or prevent these milestones from progressing in a regular pattern. This chapter provides an overview of the multifactorial influences on adolescent physical development. Psychological development is discussed in chapter 4. More concise and extensive reviews are listed in the reference section for those who want more detailed information.

Longitudinal and cross-sectional studies over the last hundred years have revealed, in the United States, an increase in height averaging 1 inch every 25 years for both sexes. Menarche has occurred earlier with each generation, such that in the United States the average adolescent will begin to menstruate during the 12th year, almost 5 years sooner than adolescents did 100 years ago (Daniel, 1970). The causes for these earlier pubertal changes are multiple, but certainly nutritional, environmental, and genetic factors have been of paramount importance.

Growth changes usually occur in the same sequence with considerable variation in the time of onset, and the amount and velocity at which they occur (Tanner, 1969). Growth occurs in every organ system of the body, with only the thymus, tonsils, and adenoids showing an obvious decrease in size. Skeletal mass, heart, lungs, liver, spleen, kidneys, pancreas, thyroids, adrenals, gonads, phallus, and uterus all double in size, while the central nervous system increases minimally (Barnes, 1975).

## ENDOCRINOLOGICAL CHANGES

The onset of puberty is marked by the appearance of secondary sex characteristics that result from the trophic effects of the gonadal hormones. The endocrinology of puberty is not fully understood, but it is known that puberty is dependent on the maturation of the central nervous system and the hypothalamic-pituitary-gonadal regulatory mechanisms. During childhood, it is thought, the hypothalamic-pituitary axis is sensitive to feedback inhibition by small amounts of gonadal steroids. At puberty the hypothalamic-pituitary axis becomes "less sensitive" to the feedback control by the gonadal hormones resulting in the increased production of releasing factors from the hypothalamus. These releasing factors, in turn, stimulate the anterior pituitary gland to secrete increased amounts of gonadal trophic hormones (i.e., follicle stimulating hormone and luteinizing hormone). These two trophic hormones then stimulate production of gonadal hormones (testosterone and estrogen) which help induce puberty, along with adrenal, thyroid, and growth hormones. Figure 1 presents a simplified view of the interrelations of the endocrine system at puberty. A detailed account of the endocrinology of puberty is beyond the scope of this chapter. Excellent reviews are presented elsewhere (August, 1972, Cheek, 1974, Donaldson, 1965, Kulin, 1969).

## LINEAR GROWTH

The vast majority of increase in height for both sexes occurs during a span of 24 to 36 months that is termed the adolescent growth spurt. This spurt is characterized by an acceleration of linear growth

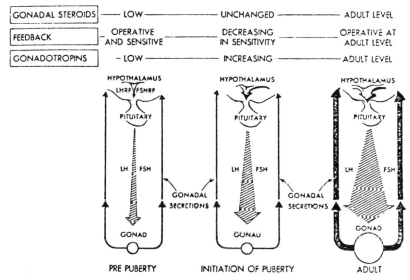

Figure 1.   Schematic diagram of the progressive change in gonadotropin secretion that results from a decrease in hypothalamic sensitivity to gonadal steroids. (Reprinted from Reiter, W. O., and Root, A. W.: Hormonal changes of adolescence. Med. Clin. N. Am. (W. B. Saunders, Philadelphia), 1975.)

velocity, a peak period of growth, which then is followed by a sharp decline in growth velocity. Growth occurs in the same fashion for both sexes but its onset averages two years earlier and slightly less in magnitude in females (Barnes, 1975, Tanner, 1962). The onset of this growth spurt varies in females between 9.5 years to 14.5 years (Figure 2); in males the onset can be between 10.5 years and 16 years (Figure 3). In females the average age of peak growth is 12.1 years, with a peak velocity of 3.25 inches per year. Ninety-nine percent of growth has occurred by age 18 (Barnes, 1975).

## MUSCLE AND FAT DISTRIBUTION

In addition to linear growth, there are major changes in both the distribution and composition of body tissues. Both sexes have similar body composition and strength prior to puberty. With the onset of the growth spurt, the rate of fat accumulation decreases significantly for females whereas males actually show an absolute loss of fat. After peak growth has occurred, adipose tissue in females is rapidly added. Males add fat tissue more slowly and less quantitatively. The greater

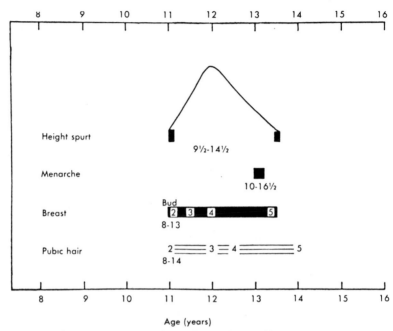

Figure 2.   Diagram of sequence of growth in girls at adolescence. An average girl is represented. The range of ages within which some of the events may occur is given by the figures placed directly below them. From: Tanner, J. M. 1962. Growth at Adolescence. (2nd ed.). Blackwell Scientific Publications, Oxford.

proportion of adipose tissue is decisive in the menstrual activity of the female. Approximately 17% body mass as fat is necessary for the onset of menstrual periods. 22% body mass as fat is needed for continuation of regular ovulatory cycles (Frisch and Revelle, 1971).

The accumulation of muscle tissue, reflected as lean body mass, is significantly greater in the male than the female after critical heights (different for each sex) have been achieved (Frisch and Revelle, 1971). Studies have shown that males not only have more muscle mass but also increased size of individual cells (Daniel, 1970). The distribution of muscle mass is significantly different with males having greater concentration of muscle in the thighs, shoulders, and back. These differences may be in response to the trophic effects of androgens, although this is far from conclusive (Daniel, 1970).

## CHANGE IN WEIGHT

On the average, the adolescent doubles his ideal body weight during puberty. The manner in which weight is added is similar to that by which linear growth is attained. There is an acceleration in velocity of weight gain, with a period of peak weight gain, followed by a decline in the velocity of weight gain. The curves reflecting weight gain are similar to those showing linear growth (Barnes, 1975). The peak period of weight gain for the female occurs six months after her period of most rapid linear growth. In the male, in contrast, the periods of peak linear growth and weight gain coincide. Thus, in contrast to linear growth where the female peaks a full 2 years before the male, the female's peak weight gain occurs only an average of 1.5 years before that of the male.

With respect to changes in both weight and height, the velocity of change may vary. However, for each individual, the patterns of growth should be consistent so that when weights and heights are plotted as a function of age, a smooth curve is obtained. Standard graphs plotting height versus age, and weight versus age are readily available and can serve as accurate assessments of the progress of puberty. For any individual, normal growth should occur along a particular

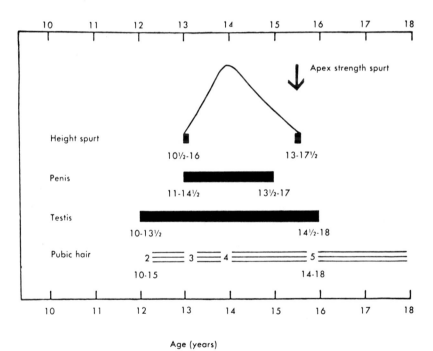

Age (years)

Figure 3. Diagram of sequence of growth in boys at adolescence. An average boy is represented. The range of ages within which each event charted may begin and end is given by the figures placed directly below its start and finish. From: Tanner, J. M. 1962. Growth at Adolescence. (2nd ed.). Blackwell Scientific Publications, Oxford.

percentile without significant variation—assuming that percentile is not below the 3rd nor above the 97th percentiles, which represent the lower and upper limits of normal, that is, $\pm 2$ S.D. from the mean (Barnes, 1975 and Kogut, 1973).

Comparison of height and weight percentiles may provide clues to the development of a disease. In general no more than a 15-percentile difference should exist in an individual's height and weight for a particular chronological age (Barnes, 1975). For example, an individual who is at the 90th percentile in weight and the 60th percentile for height is probably obese, whereas if the individual were in the 15th percentile for weight (and 60th percentile for height) evaluation for chronic malnutrition or a chronic, subclinical disease should be considered. Diseases such as juvenile rheumatoid arthritis, systemic lupus erythematosus, chronic hepatitis, hyperthyroidism, regional enteritis, and chronic urinary tract infections and undiagnosed anorexia nervosa may first be reflected in an actual decrease or plateauing of weight (Barnes, 1975, Frisch and Revelle, 1969, McCaffery et al, 1970, Sopel and Stolz, 1962). To reiterate, the key to assessing "normalcy" of changes in both height and weight lies in accurate records of the adolescent's growth curves with respect to both the onset of the growth spurt and the patient's progression through the various stages (Tanner, 1962, 1966).

## SEXUAL MATURATION

The hallmark of adolescence, discounting the growth spurt, is the development of secondary sexual characteristics, which for females includes the onset of menarche. Intimately related to these profound physical changes is much of the emotional turmoil that so characteristically engulfs the changing adolescent. The adolescent, during the period of rapid bodily changes, is constantly comparing himself to his peers. This can be fraught with misgivings at the least, or with serious concerns about inadequacy or abnormality in its extreme. The professional who is actively involved with adolescents and who is at all sensitive, realizes this intuitively. To realistically help the adolescent with his concerns, however, an intimate knowledge of the stages of sexual development, and the allowable degrees of variation, is mandatory. To that end, Tanner's criteria (Marshall and Tanner, 1969) provide a descriptive maturational framework by which objective assessment of sexual growth can be understood and followed. The adolescent's stage of pubertal development should be checked at each visit so that abnormalities may be noted and explored (Barnes, 1975). More important, reassurances to the adolescent that development is proceeding normally may provide crucial support to the adolescent who harbors "unspeakable" concerns about his body. The Tanner stages for females and males are given in Tables 1 and 2. (For comparisons with growth refer to Figures 2 and 3).

Secondary sexual development in the female begins with the development of breast buds and/or the growth of pubic hair. According to Tanner's data, the mean ages for both are 11.2 years (B-2) and 11.7 years (PH-2) respectively (Marshall and Tanner, 1969). Despite these close means, however, it is important to realize that the correlation between breast development and pubic hair growth is variable. The initial onset of each, as well as the rapidity with which each stage is reached is also variable (Marshall and Tanner, 1969).

Despite these variations in development, several definitive statements can be made. Using the mean ages for breast bud and pubic hair growth given above and defining normalcy as $\pm 2$ S.D. (i.e., 2.2 years and 2.4 years, respectively), then it follows that patients with breast development (B-2) before 9 years should be assessed for premature thelarche if no pubic hair is present (Silver and Sami, 1968). Those with pubic hair growth (PH-2) before 9.3 years should be evaluated for premature pubarche (Barnes, 1975, Silverman et al, 1952). Conversely, assessment for delayed puberty should be considered if breast development (B-2) is delayed beyond 13.4 years or if the growth of pubic hair (PH-2) does not occur before 14.1 years (Barnes, 1975, Marshall and Tanner, 1969, Reiter, 1972). Other extensive correlations between the various stages of breast and pubic hair growth have been made by Barnes.

Table 1.   Classification of sex maturity stages in girls

| Stage | Pubic hair | Breasts |
|---|---|---|
| 1 | Preadolescent | Preadolescent |
| 2 | Sparse, lightly pigmented, straight, medial border of labia | Breast and papilla elevated as small mound; areolar diameter increased |
| 3 | Darker, beginning to curl, increased amount | Breast and areola enlarged, no contour separation |
| 4 | Coarse, curly, abundant but amount less than in adult | Areola and papilla form secondary mound |
| 5 | Adult feminine triangle, spread to medial surface of thighs | Mature; nipple projects, areola part of general breast contour |

From: Daniel, U. A. 1970. The Adolescent Patient. C. V. Mosby, St. Louis.

Table 2.   Classification of genitalia maturity stages in boys

| Stage | Pubic hair | Penis | Testes |
|---|---|---|---|
| 1 | None | Preadolescent | |
| 2 | Slight, long, slightly pigmented | Slight enlargement | Enlarged scrotum, pink, texture altered |
| 3 | Darker, starts to curl, small amount | Penis longer | Larger |
| 4 | Resembles adult type, but less in quantity, coarse, curly | Larger, glans and breadth increase in size | Larger, scrotum dark |
| 5 | Adult distribution spread to medial surface of thighs | Adult | Adult |

From: Daniel, U. A. 1970. The Adolescent Patient. C. V. Mosby, St. Louis.

The descriptions of the various stages are presented in Table 1. The figures are concise and provide the professional with a means to classify any females that are evaluated.

Menarche most commonly begins when most (60%) of females are at a stage of B-4 breast development, which coincides to mean chronical age of 12.7 years (Marshall and Tanner, 1969). Ninety-nine percent of females will have onset of menarche within 5 years of breast budding (B-2). As already mentioned, the onset of menses is closely correlated with the percent of body fat. To reiterate, 17% body fat is needed for initiation of menses, while 22% body fat is necessary for sustaining regular menstrual periods (Frisch and Revelle, 1971). This is also the period of maximal weight gain in the adolescent female (see Figure 2).

Menstrual cycles are commonly irregular for the first several months and then often become relatively predictable. According to Zacharis and Wurtman (1969), the mean age for onset of regular menses is 13.8 $\pm$2 years. Thus, in the absence of associated symptoms, patients with irregular menstrual periods of less than 2 years duration should be reassured. Those with irregular menses for longer than 2 years should have a full gynecological assessment (Barnes, 1975).

Menarche before 10.3 years (12.7 $\pm$2 S.D.) should be considered premature and should be evaluated. Conversely the patient who hasn't had the onset of menses by age 15.5, assuming other parameters of growth and sexual maturation are normal, should be evaluated for primary amenorrhea.

The development of secondary sexual changes in the male follows comparable sequential stages descriptively outlined by Tanner and presented in Table 2. Male pubertal development is initiated by scrotal and testicular enlargement (G-2) with a mean age of onset being 11.6 ±1 year (Marshall and Tanner, 1969). Using 2 S.D. as the criteria for statistical normalcy, it follows that those males with onset or G-2 before 9.5 years or after 13.6 years should be evaluated for precocious puberty and delayed puberty respectively (Barnes, 1975, Marshall and Tanner, 1970, Stolz and Stolz, 1951).

As in female development, male genital and pubic hair development occur sequentially. However, the correlations between them varies, as do both the time of onset and the speed with which each stage is attained. Each should thus be staged separately (Barnes, 1975, Marshall and Tanner, 1970). The average time between onset of scrotal/testicular enlargement and completion of genital development is 3.3 years (mean age 14.9 ±1.1 S.D.), (Marshall and Tanner, 1970).

About 75% of males will have their maximal growth during G-4, as shown in Figure 3. This is comparable to females' maximal growth during B-4 described in Figure 2. Although there is a great deal of individual variation, generally, axillary hair appears approximately two years after pubic hair (PH) growth begins, facial hair begins during late PH-3 and reaches adult distribution by PH-5 (Barnes, 1975, Marshall and Tanner, 1970).

Stimulation of male breast development may occur in almost 30% of normal adolescents, resulting in 80% of cases having nontender, bilateral gynecomastia. About 20% of these males may have unilateral and/or tender breast masses (Barnes, 1975). Reassurance that they are normal in males may help greatly in alleviating anxiety associated with such a development. The gynecomastia, which can develop rapidly over a period of several months, may require over a year for resolution. It is suggested that breast tissue that is persistent beyond 18 months after its appearance or which severely disturbs the adolescent male should be surgically removed. Rarely is adolescent gynecomastia pathological (Barnes, 1975, Gallagher and Heald, 1976, Wilkins, 1948).

## THE ADOLESCENT WITH DEVELOPMENTAL DISABILITIES

Although puberty does vary significantly in onset, progression, and completion, it has been pointed out that adolescent growth occurs in stages. Adolescents complete these stages in a sequential fashion. This is an important concept to remember as one approaches health care of the developmentally disabled adolescent. Depending on the handicap, completion of growth and development may be delayed, altered or inhibited. In such cases, therefore, health care will vary significantly both in content and delivery. For example, the 15-year-old moderately retarded, sexually active female will require a significantly different approach to discussing contraception and hygiene. Likewise the 18-year-old male with significant deficits resulting from cerebral palsy will need assistance in defining and working toward a vocational objective.

Throughout this chapter emphasis has been on the adolescents' physical maturation. The psychological reactions to these tremendous physical changes can be varied and enormous as Dr. Katz points out in chapter 4. Nurses involved with the developmentally disabled adolescent should note that development is always accompanied by psychological reactions to these changes. When physical disabilities are present, aberrant and/or abnormal emotional growth may also occur. The 14-year-old male with grand mal seizures, if not well controlled with anticonvulsants, must live with restrictions on his participation in athletics and extracurricular activities. His feelings of self-esteem and physical control of his body will deviate widely from that experienced by his companion who has no similar problem. His constant anxiety concerning convulsions, with their notable concomitants like soiling, may lead to regressive behavior and/or delayed emotional growth.

## CONCLUSION

The combinations of physical and pyschological alterations that may develop in a developmentally disabled adolescent are many. Recognition of these abnormal developments and effective intervention to prevent or minimize their results is possible only if those changes are noted. It is incumbant upon health care practitioners that they remain sensitized to the special needs of developmentally disabled adolescents. Understanding normal maturation is a necessity for that sensitivity and for providing comprehensive health care.

## REFERENCES CITED

August, G. P., et al. 1972. Hormonal changes in puberty. III. correlation of plasma testosterone, LH, FSH, testicular size, an bone age with male pubertal developments. J. Clin. Endocrinol. Metab. 34:319.

Barker, P. G., Wright, B. A., and Gonick, M. A. 1953. Adjustment to physical handicap and illness: A survey of the social psychology of physique and disability. Social Science Research Council Bulletin 55, (revised), Social Science Research Council, New York.

Barnes, H. U. 1975. Physical growth and development during puberty. Med. Clin. N. Am. 59:6:1305.

Battle, C. U. 1975. Chronic physical disease. Pediatr. Clin. N. Am. 22:525.

Castlle, G. F., and Fishman, L. S. 1973. Seizures. Pediatr. Clin. N. Am. 20:819.

Cheek, D. B. 1968. Human Growth: Body Composition, Cell Growth, Energy, and Intelligence. Lea and Febiger, Philadelphia.

Cheek, D. B. 1974. Body composition, hormones, nutrition and adolescent growth. In: M. M. Grumbach, C. D. Grave, and F. E. Mauer. (eds.), Control of the Onset of Puberty. John Wiley & Sons. New York.

Daniel, W. A. 1970. The Adolescent Patient. C. V. Mosby, St. Louis.

Donovan, B. T., and Van Der Werff Ten Bosch, J. J. 1965. Physiology of Puberty. Williams & Wilkins, Baltimore.

Frisch, R. E., and Revelle, R. 1969. The height and weight of adolescent boys and girls at the time of peak velocity in height and weight: longitudinal data. Human Biol. 41:526.

Frisch, R. E., and Revelle, R. 1971a. The height and weight of girls and boys at the time of initiation of the adolescent growth spurt in height and weight. Human Biol. 43:140.

Frisch, R. E., and Revelle, R. 1971b. Height and weight at menarche, and a hypothesis of menarche. Arch. Dis. Child. 46:695.

Gallagher, J. R., Heald, F. P., Garell, D. C. 1976. Medical Care of the Adolescent (3rd ed.). Appleton-Century-Crofts, New York.

Hall, J. E. 1974. Sexual Behavior. In: J. Worts, (ed.), Mental Retardation and Development Disabilities (UI). Brunner/Mazel, New York.

Heald, F. P. 1968. Anatomy, physiology, and pharmacology (of the adolescent). In: Cooke, R. E., The Biologic Basis of Pediatric Practice, Vol. 2. McGraw-Hill, New York.

Kogut, M. D. 1973. Growth and development in adolescence. Pediatr. Clin. N. Am. 20:4:789.

Kulin, H. E., Grumbach, M. M., and Kaplan, S. L. 1969. Changing sensitivity of the pubertal gonadal hypothalamic feedback mechanism in man. Science 166:1012.

Marshall, W. A., and Tanner, J. M. 1969. Variations in patterns of pubertal changes in girls. Arch. Dis. Child. 44:291.

Marshall, W. A., and Tanner, J. M. 1970. Variations in patterns of pubertal changes in boys. Arch. Dis. Child. 45:13.

McCaffery, T. D., Nasr, K., Lawrence, A. M., et al. 1970. Severe growth retardation in children with inflammatory bowel disease. Pediatrics 45:386.

Reiter, E. O., Kulin, H. E. 1972. Sexual maturation in the female, Pediatr. Clin. N. Am. 19(3):581.

Schonfeld, W. A. 1943. Primary and secondary sexual characteristics. Am. J. Dis. Child. 65:535.

Silver, H. K., and Sami, D. 1968. Premature thelarche: precocious development of the breast. Pediatrics 34:107.

Silverman, S. H., et al. 1952. Precocious growth of sexual hair without other secondary sexual development: Premature pubarche a constitutional variation of adolescence. Pediatrics 10:426.

Stolz, H. R. and Stolz, L. M. 1951. Somatic Development of Adolescent Boys. Macmillan, New York.

Sobel, E. H., Silverman, F. N., and Lee, C. M., Jr. 1962. Chronic regional enteritis and growth retardation. Am. J. Dis. Child. 103:569.

Tanner, J. M. 1962. Growth at Adolescence. (2nd ed.). Blackwell Scientific, Oxford.

Tanner, J. M., and Whitehouse, R. H. 1966. Growth and Development Record, BHWU 13 and 14.

Tanner, J. M., et al. 1966. Standards from birth to maturity for height, weight, height velocity, weight velocity: British children, 1965. Part I and II, Arch. Dis. Child. 41:454, 613.

Usdane, W. M. 1974. Vocational planning for the handicapped adolescent. In: J. A. Downey, and N. L. Law. (eds.), The Child With Disabling Illness. W. B. Saunders, Philadelphia.

Wilkins, L. 1948. Abnormalities and variations in sexual development during childhood and adolescence. Adv. Pediat. 3:159.

Zacharias, L., and Wurtman, R. J. 1969. Age at menarche, N. Engl. J. Med. 280:868.

Zacharias, L., and Wurtman, R. J., et al. 1970. Sexual maturation in contemporary American girls. Am. J. Obstet. Gynec. 108:833.

# chapter four

# PSYCHOLOGICAL CONCEPTS

Kathy S. Katz, Ph.D.

## DEVELOPMENTAL TASKS OF ADOLESCENCE

### Normal Adolescent Development

Adolescence is felt to be a time in which even normal individuals experience a period of crisis marked by conflict and rebellion. Many psychologists have felt that this period of turmoil is a necessary part of the process of maturing (Kiell, 1964).

The belief that adolescence is a time of storm and strife has an important place in psychoanalytic theory. Anna Freud's (1964) list of the developmental tasks of adolescence includes proper control and expression of increased sexual and aggressive desires, and changes in the relationships with parents and peer group. Because of the intensity of the desires experienced in adolescence, Freud views conflict and upheaval as unavoidable for the individual during this period.

Erik Erikson (1950) in his book on the eight stages of man, describes the advent of puberty as the beginning of the stage of "identity versus role confusion." The adolescent becomes concerned about how he appears to others and about how he feels about himself. Though the youth is experiencing enormous physiological changes, he seeks to connect the feelings about himself developed during childhood with the maturing individual that others now regard him as being. If the adolescent is able to integrate what he has been in the past with his current meaning to others, he achieves a sense of ego identity. While the formation of one's identity is really a process that continues throughout life, in our culture it becomes a focal task during adolescence. For the adolescent who has difficulty forming an ego identity, the result is role confusion. Often it is the inability to settle on an occupational identity, according to Erikson, which disturbs young people. The need to appear the same as peers and to exclude those that are different is viewed as a defense against a sense of identity confusion.

As the adolescent emerges into young adulthood he moves into Erikson's stage of Intimacy versus Isolation. The young person is ready to fuse his identity with that of others. In so doing, he commits himself to certain affiliations that may require him at times to make personal sacrifices and compromises. If the young person cannot make these affiliations because of fears of loss of his own identity, a sense of isolation results.

In summary, the most important of the developmental tasks for the adolescent center on learning to handle sexual and aggressive impulses, formation of an independent ego identity, and eventually, formation of intimate relationships with others.

## Psychosocial Development of the Developmentally Disabled

The psychosocial development of the developmentally disabled adolescent depends to a large extent on his degree of cognitive deficit. The individual's level of cognitive functioning generally determines his level of psychosocial development. His ability to function autonomously and to form relationships with others usually corresponds closely with his level of cognitive abilities.

The milder the degree of cognitive deficit, the more closely one would expect the development of the developmentally disabled adolescent to follow that of the normal adolescent. The majority of the more severely retarded will never reach what would correspond to the adolescent level of psychosocial functioning in the normal individual.

As noted by de la Cruz and La Veck (1973), the adolescent period for the mildly developmentally disabled individual follows much the same course as that of the normal individual only it occurs at a later chronological age. The mildly impaired youth also struggles for self-identification and a mature sex role preference, but he achieves these things at a later age than the normal adolescent. The mildly retarded individual shows as much interest in heterosexuals as the normal adolescent. The majority of the severely retarded, however, show no interest in the opposite sex at maturity.

## LEVEL OF COGNITION AND EXPECTATIONS
## FOR DEVELOPMENTALLY DISABLED ADOLESCENTS

Knowledge of the individual's degree of cognitive deficit is necessary in order to determine at what level of psychosocial functioning he might be capable of performing. Cognition is usually described in terms of the retardation classification used by the American Association on Mental Deficiency (Table 1).

### Determining Level of Cognitive Function

Two major areas of functioning are considered in determining the individual's level of functioning. The first of these is the level of cognitive functioning as measured by administration of one or more standardized intelligence tests. Also necessary in making any statement about the level of retardation, however, is some measure of the individual's social adaptive functioning (see chapter 2 for discussion of adaptive functioning). This would entail assessment of the adolescent's self-help skills and his degree of independent functioning. These skills require practical judgment and common sense learning which are quite different than the abilities measured by intelligence tests. Adaptive functioning is also more affected by the training the individual has received than are cognitive abilities. It is quite common to see retarded persons whose adaptive functioning is a good deal higher than one would expect on the basis of scores achieved on cognitive tests. In such a case the individual's actual functioning level would have to be considered in the light of the strengths he demonstrated in adaptive skills. This may have different implications in vocational planning than if decisions were made on the basis of measured IQ alone.

Table 1.   American Association of Mental Deficiency classification of mental retardation

|  | Standard deviation | Wechsler IQ score | Binet IQ score |
|---|---|---|---|
| Mildly retarded | 3 below the mean | 55–69 | 52–67 |
| Moderately retarded | 4 below the mean | 40–54 | 36–51 |
| Severely retarded | 5 below the mean | 25–39 | 20–35 |
| Profoundly retarded | 6 below the mean | Below 25 | Below 20 |

## Criticism of Intelligence Testing

In recent years, intelligence tests have been the subject of much criticism. These tests were developed initially to assist in predicting academic performance among school-age children, and they remain the best tool we have for predicting academic achievement. When used with developmentally disabled individuals, the IQ test can help in planning a school program that would be most suitable for that child. Certain expectations can be set for a child of a given level of cognitive functioning.

## The Mildly Retarded Adolescent

*Educational Expectations*   According to the AAMD classification the mildly retarded child is one who achieves an IQ score in the range of 55 to 69 (an IQ of 100 is considered the average score). The mildly retarded child would require special education services throughout elementary school and perhaps throughout most of secondary school as well. The mildly retarded child is considered to be educable; that is, he can be expected to achieve at least basic reading and arithmetic skills perhaps up to a 3rd or 4th grade level. Class placement, depending on the individual school system, might range from a self-contained classroom for educable mentally retarded children to a primarily mainstreamed program with participation in a resource program for major academic subjects.

*Vocational Expectations*   As the mildly retarded child moves into adolescence, the focus of his school program generally shifts from academic to vocational training. Around ages 16 to 18 the typical developmentally disabled individual has reached his maximal level of academic achievement. It is at this age that cognitive development reaches a plateau. Adaptive skills may continue to develop, however. The individual continues to have the ability to learn new skills well into adulthood.

With the proper vocational training the majority of mildly retarded individuals are employable and, for the most part, capable of independent living. Many could be capable of joining the work force and living a life largely indistinguishable from that of the normal population.

## The Moderately Retarded Adolescent

*Educational Expectations*   The moderately retarded individual is one who achieves an IQ score in the range of 40 to 54. These individuals are considered to be trainable. Their educational program generally takes place in a self-contained special education classroom where the focus is on the development of maximal self-help and independence skills. Reading skills for this group of developmentally disabled individuals are generally limited to recognizing important words and signs. Arithmetic skills usually do not go beyond some basic counting skills.

*Vocational Expectations*   In the adolescent years, focus for the moderately retarded individual is on development of skills necessary for participation in some structured employment situation, most often a sheltered workshop program. Many moderately retarded persons have the ability to perform a variety of manipulative tasks if given specialized training. They may continue to need more support and supervision however, than is generally provided in the usual employment situation.

## Residential Alternatives for Mildly and Moderately Retarded Adults

While some mildly retarded individuals often are capable of independent living, many mildly retarded and the majority of moderately retarded persons require some type of supervision and guidance in their living situation. This need not necessarily be in the parental home, and it certainly need not be in a large institutional setting.

*The Community Residence*   There are a growing number of community group homes for developmentally disabled older adolescents and adults. This residence is usually a house or apartment building in the community with one or more normal adults who oversee the running of the house. The retarded residents participate in house management and often are employed outside the residence. The group home arrangement allows a much greater degree of autonomous functioning than developmentally disabled individuals were allowed to assume in the past, though many were capable of it. Thus the community residence allows the maintenance and establishment of behaviors that are as culturally normative as possible (Wolfensberger, 1972).

In a study of the behavior shown by developmentally disabled residents in a community group home, Nihira and Nihira (1975) observed that the residents gained in skills such as cleaning and maintaining their rooms, bed making, ironing, simple food preparation, and yard work. Many of the house residents learned to move about the community safely and independently. Many were noted to improve in eating skills, verbal communication, and in handling simple economic tasks.

*Implications of Residence Living for Psychosocial Development In Developmentally Disabled Persons*    The development of facilities for retarded individuals such as community residences has had important implications for the psychological development of the developmentally disabled adolescent. As noted earlier in the chapter, one of the major developmental tasks of adolescence is the development of an independent identity. Opportunities for independent functioning had been very limited for the developmentally disabled adolescent in the past. If living in his parents' home, he continued in a child role indefinitely. Parents of handicapped individuals have been found to be overprotective of their children and have not allowed their children to function as autonomously as they were often capable of doing (Bell, 1964). Thus the developmentally disabled adolescent was denied the opportunities given to normal adolescents, to separate and to begin to form an independent identity. King (1971) notes that the adolescent period may be less tumultuous if certain social conditions exist that allow the individual to achieve his mature identity without undue stress. Among these conditions is the existence of meaningful adult roles that bring with them rewards for their fulfillment. Another important condition is the clear definition of transition points from child to adult status. Community residences can now provide these necessary transition points for the developmentally disabled individual.

## Marital Relationships for Developmentally Disabled Adults

Moving into adulthood, the goal for many mildly retarded individuals, and perhaps even some of those moderately retarded, is an eventual marital relationship. Studies by Flour et al (1975) and Berry and Shapiro (1975) have investigated the marital adjustment of developmentally disabled young adults. Both studies noted similar characteristics in their groups. Both studies found a low rate of divorce or separation among the couples. Those couples that chose to have children usually had no more than two. Child care was found to be adequate in almost all cases. Work records among the individuals were highly satisfactory although at times of stress they were more subject to periods of absenteeism. Marital conflict tended to center around problems of money management, indebtedness, and demanding relatives. Most couples continued to need support and guidance from social agencies or families. Flour et al suggest that training be provided in budgeting and money management, sex education, premarital counseling and contraceptive information, for developmentally disabled couples considering marriage.

For those developmentally disabled couples who plan to have children, the prognosis seems to be good that these children will have normal functioning. Laxova et al (1973) found that mothers who themselves had nonspecific subnormality had a high percentage of children with normal IQ's.

### Expectations for Severely and Profoundly Retarded Persons

Severely retarded individuals, those with IQ's in the range of 25 to 39, and the profoundly retarded, with IQ's below 25 will be in need of supervision throughout their lifetimes. Most developmentally disabled adolescents at this level of functioning are not considered trainable in terms of vocational skills. Many, however, are capable of varying degrees of self-care under supervision. The goals for severely and profoundly retarded individuals are to maximize self help skills in toileting, self-feeding and dressing. Facilities exist in many communities to provide weekly recreational programs for the severely developmentally disabled that offer opportunities for peer contact and activity. If adequate community support services exist, many of these individuals can remain with their families and may not require institutional placement.


### PSYCHOLOGICAL ASSESSMENT

As mentioned previously, in order to determine appropriate expectations for a developmentally disabled person, his level of cognitive and adaptive functioning must be assessed. This assessment is usually in the form of psychological testing.

### Intellectual Assessment

In determining the level of cognitive functioning, the test used is the intelligence scale which yields an Intelligence Quotient (IQ) score. The IQ was originally conceived as a measure of the individual's mental age relative to his chronological age, with the IQ score being a ratio of these two numbers. Thus if a person's mental age level was the same as his chronological age, he was considered average and the IQ score ratio was given as 100.

The IQ tests most commonly used with adolescents are the Wechsler Intelligence Scale for Children-Revised (WISC-R), the Wechsler Adult Intelligence Scale (WAIS), the Stanford-Binet, and the Columbia Mental Maturity Scale. These tests were originally developed in an attempt to predict academic achievement. Intended as tests of scholastic aptitude rather than as tests of general learning, the standardized intelligence tests may not adequately assess the retarded adolescent's ability. Specific deficits in language or motor functioning may also make valid evaluation of test scores difficult. The psychologist should attempt in these cases to use the test that is best geared to evaluate the individual's areas of strength.

The intelligence test will, however, give one a general range to consider in terms of cognitive functioning. This must then be considered in conjunction with objective measures of the individual's adaptive, or practical skills. Tests frequently used to measure these skills are the Vineland Scale of Social Maturity and the Adaptive Behavior Rating Scale. Items on these scales measure abilities such as feeding and dressing skills and other behavior related to independent functioning. (See chapter 2 for further discussion of adaptive skills.) Measures of this type enable us to evaluate how the individual functions in day to day activities. His level of overall cognitive functioning is thus determined with both intellectual and adaptive skills taken into account.

**Perceptual Motor Assessment**

Another area of cognitive functioning that is often assessed by the psychologist and may be useful in terms of vocational planning is the area of perceptual motor or visual motor functioning. This skill requires the individual to analyze a problem visually and then to coordinate his hands with his eyes to carry out the task. One test used by psychologists to measure visual motor functioning is the Bender-Gestalt test. This test requires the individual to copy a series of geometric designs and then to reproduce some of them from memory. Measurement of this skill can be important in vocational planning because if an individual shows marked deficits in this area, he will likely encounter difficulty in a job that requires a good deal of manual dexterity.

**Vocational Assessment**

Further assessment may be needed in the areas of vocationally applicable skills. These skills actually may play a more important part in planning for the developmentally disabled adolescent than more purely intellectual skills which are more geared to educational prediction. (see chapter 10 for a discussion of vocational assessments and planning.)

**Personality Assessment**

In addition to assessing cognitive functioning, a psychologist can also evaluate personality functioning (Exner, 1976). Psychological tests, called projective tests, have been developed to allow the psychologist to determine areas of emotional concern for the individual. These tests are usually administered to people who are referred for evaluation because of difficulties in social or emotional functioning. These personality tests are called "projective" tests because the person projects his own feelings through verbal responses to a set of standardized cards. The psychologist then makes interpretations from the themes expressed in the responses, as to what the person's emotional concerns might be.

The intent is that given the ambiguous quality of the stimulus cards of the projective tests, the person will express his particular personality traits and emotional response tendencies. From this information the psychologist can suggest what kind of intervention might be helpful in alleviating the difficulties the person is experiencing.

The projective tests most frequently used in the adolescent period are the Rorschach Inkblot Test and the Thematic Apperception Test (TAT).

*The Rorschach Test*    The Rorschach test consists of a series of 10 inkblots to which the person must respond giving his interpretation of each blot. This test can be useful in determining when an individual's perceptions differ from those of others, implying disturbance in reality testing. The test is thus often used in diagnosing psychotic disturbance.

*The Thematic Apperception Test*    The TAT consists of a series of pictures many of which depict people in a variety of ambiguous situations. The individual is asked to make up a story about what is happening in the picture, how the people feel, and what the outcome is.

*Use of Projective Tests With Developmentally Disabled Persons* Because the projective tests described require verbal responses, verbal expressive ability must be present in order to obtain usable results from these tests. The individual tested must have a high enough level of verbal conceptualization to do more than merely list items he sees in the TAT cards, for example. In using projective testing with developmentally disabled adolescents, their level of verbal conceptualization must be kept in mind. Use of tests of this type would most probably be limited to developmentally disabled individuals who have mild or moderate levels of retardation with mental ages of at least 7 or 8 years. Even at this mental age level, some retarded individuals may have a concrete level of conceptualization and it may be difficult for them to understand the more abstract concepts of time and emotion.

### Behavioral Assessment

Another technique for evaluation of disturbances in emotional functioning is behavioral assessment. This technique can be used with developmentally disabled individuals of all levels of retardation, including those at the severe and profound level.

*Principle of Behavioral Assessment*   The basic principle in the behavioral approach to assessing personality disturbance is that the individual is somehow receiving an unintentional reward for the undesirable behavior he is demonstrating (Goldfried, 1976). For instance, a profoundly retarded individual in an institutional setting may attract the attention of the caretakers because of disruptive behavior. The developmentally disabled individual likes getting attention but when he is behaving well no one pays attention to him. Thus the disruptive behavior can get him a reward (attention) that he does not ordinarily receive.

*Implementing a Behavioral Assessment*   To correct behavioral problems, what is needed is an assessment of what conditions in the individual's environment are rewarding the undesirable behavior. Additionally, an assessment must be made of what kinds of new rewards can be built into the individual's daily experience to encourage the development of more adaptive behaviors. The psychologist performing the assessment gathers baseline data by observing the individual in the situations where the problems are occurring, recording what environmental events preceded and followed the problem behavior, and noting how often the specified behavior occurred. The psychologist carefully observes how other individuals in the developmentally disabled person's environment interact with him to discover how their behavior might be influencing his.

## THERAPEUTIC INTERVENTION

When certain behavioral or emotional problems have been identified in a developmentally disabled adolescent, the next question is what to do about them. A variety of psychotherapeutic techniques can be employed to effect a behavior or personality change to bring about better adjustment in the individual.

Psychotherapy may generally be defined as "the systematic utilization of psychological techniques chief of which is a close interpersonal relationship by a professionally trained therapist in order to help individuals who need or seek his assistance in the amelioration of their emotional problems. The procedures involved may include nonverbal as well as verbal techniques and the subjects may or may not be aware of the dynamics of the therapeutic process" (Bialer, 1967).

## Insight Model of Psychotherapy

One type of psychotherapeutic approach is the "insight" model. In this type of treatment the individual discusses his thoughts and feelings with his therapist. The therapist first helps him in interpreting what feelings motivate his behavior, and then helps him in resolving conflicts that may be interfering with his emotional functioning. This type of treatment requires verbal conceptualization ability, and so it is most often limited to mildly or moderately mentally retarded individuals. For persons with cerebral palsy or other disorders where verbal expression is difficult, alternative means of expressing feelings may be used. Through work with clay or painting the individual can communicate his feelings to his therapist, who in turn can help interpret those feelings and help the developmentally disabled person better understand his problems.

Insight psychotherapy is most often provided by professionals trained in understanding personality dynamics. This might be a psychiatrist, psychologist, social worker, or psychiatric nurse.

## Group Approaches to Insight Psychotherapy

Insight psychotherapy can also involve a group therapy model. In this treatment model, a small group of individuals meets regularly under the supervision of a therapist, and the individuals within the group talk about thoughts and feelings. Other group members, in conjunction with the therapist, help the individual in understanding these feelings and may themselves better understand their own problems in learning about those of another person.

Both individual and group treatment models can be very helpful for the developmentally disabled individual during adolescence if he has adequate verbal skills. As mentioned previously, the adolescent period is an extremely stressful time for the normal and developmentally disabled adolescent alike. Psychotherapy can provide the support that the developmentally disabled adolescent needs in helping him to see his own competencies and achieve individual identity and separation from his family.

### Behavior Therapy

Behavior therapy is the treatment approach most often used with developmentally disabled individuals without the verbal skills necessary for "talking" therapies. The basic premise of this approach is that inappropriate behaviors are learned and can be unlearned. This approach does not deal with possible underlying conflicts but focuses on the undesirable behavior directly.

*Uses for Behavior Therapy* This type of approach can be extremely useful in dealing with problem areas such as toilet training and other self-care skills, temper tantrums, and social behaviors (Magrab, 1976).

As mentioned in the discussion of behavioral assessment, the behavior modifier views behavior as resulting from reinforcement. In order to correct undesirable behavior, the therapist must first identify the target behaviors. Next, he decides on appropriate reinforcement, and then he develops a reinforcement schedule to eliminate the undesirable behavior while reinforcing more adaptive ones. The desired behavior may not be a part of the developmentally disabled individual's repertoire at the beginning of treatment and in order to develop that particular behavior a process known as "shaping" is used. In shaping, behaviors that gradually approximate the desired behavior are successively reinforced.

*Use of the Shaping Technique* The shaping technique is especially effective in developing self-help skills. For example, in teaching an individual to put on his own pants, the therapist would perhaps begin by putting the pants on the person but pulling them up only to mid thigh. The developmentally disabled person would then be rewarded for pulling them up the rest of the way to his waist. Next the therapist would pull the pants up to the knee and reward the individual for completing the task from there. By use of successive approximations one could eventually have the developmentally disabled person putting on his pants entirely on his own.

In using an approach of this type, developmentally disabled individuals have been taught self-care skills such as washing, dressing and eating, vocational skills, and better language skills.

*The Token Economy*  A technique called a token economy has been found to be a useful behavior modifier in settings such as community group residences, sheltered workshops and training schools. In this system, points or chips are awarded to individuals for demonstrating certain desired behaviors. Points may be lost for such things as disruptive behavior or inattention. After acquiring a certain number of points, the developmentally disabled individual can "cash" these in for some other tangible reward or privilege.

*Implications of Behavior Therapy for the Developmentally Disabled*  Systematic behavior modification has been a tremendous advance in the treatment of the developmentally disabled. It has offered many new avenues in developing greater levels of independent functioning for those developmentally disabled individuals who were considered below the "trainable" level. Use of this treatment has done much to support the belief that even the very severely retarded individual can be taught skills that enable him to lead a more meaningful and independent life.

## REFERENCES CITED

Bell, R. 1964. The family and limited coping ability in the child. Merrill-Palmer Quart. 10:129.

Berry, J. and Shapiro, A. 1975. Married mentally handicapped patients in the community. Proc. Royal Soc. Med. 68:795–798.

Bialer, I. 1967. Psychotherapy and Other Adjustment Techniques with the Mentally Retarded. In: A. Baumeister (ed.), Mental Retardation pp. 138–180. Aldine, Chicago.

de la Cruz, F., and La Veck, G. (eds.) 1973. Human Sexuality and the Mentally Retarded. Brunner/Mazel, New York.

Erikson, E. 1950. Childhood and Society, Norton, New York.

Exner, J. 1976. Projective Techniques. In: Weiner, I. (ed.), Clinical Methods in Psychology, pp. 61–121. John Wiley & Sons, New York.

Flour, L., Baxter, D., Rosen, M., and Zisfern, L. 1975. A survey of marriages among previously institutionalized retardates. Ment. Retard. 13:33–37.

Freud, A. 1969. Adolescence as a developmental disturbance. In: G. Kaplan and S. Lebovici (eds.), Adolescence, Psychosocial Perspectives. Basic Books, New York.

Gardner, W. 1971. Behavior Modification in Mental Retardation. Aldine, Chicago.

Goldfried, M. 1976. Behavioral Assessment. In: Weiner, I. (ed.), Clinical Methods in Psychology, pp. 281–330. John Wiley & Sons, New York.

Kiell, N. 1964. The Universal Experience of Adolescence. International University Press, New York.

King, S. 1971. Coping mechanisms in adolescents. Psychiatr. Ann. 1:10–46.

Laxova, R., Gilderdale, S., and Ridler, M. 1973. An etiological study of 53 female patients from a subnormality hospital and of their offspring. J. Ment. Def. 17:193–225.

Magrab, P. 1976. Psychology. In: R. Johnston, and P. Magrab (eds.), Developmental Disorders: Assessment, Treatment, Education, pp. 207–231. University Park Press, Baltimore.

Nihira, L. and Nihira, K. 1975. Normalized behavior in community placement. Ment. Retard. 13:9–13.

Wolfensberger, W. 1972. The Principle of Normalization in Human Services. University of York Press, Toronto.

# chapter five

# THE ADOLESCENT AND THE FAMILY

Inta Adamovics Rutins, M.S.W., ACSW

The developmentally disabled adolescent, like any other human being, cannot be viewed in isolation. He is a member of a family and thus a part of a complicated system of social roles and interactions that have evolved from birth and grown more complex by adolescence. Hill (1968) defines the family as a small group, organized into paired positions of husband-father, wife-mother, son-brother, and sister-daughter. This group of personalities represents the nuclear family. Each family member interacts with every other family member. The behavior of one family member can elicit and affect the behavior of other family members. Consequently, the problem of a developmentally disabled individual must always be thought of as a family problem and considered in light of the total family situation. One must take into account the influence of the developmental disability, sociocultural factors, and service delivery system on the total family function.

The concept of the family as a unit of service has been a well established notion in nursing practice, particularly with the developmentally disabled infant and child. During adolescence nurses have many opportunities available to facilitate the teenager's independence and to help promote healthier family growth and interaction in the process. Consequently, the principal focus of this chapter will be the family viewed as the unit of treatment. Responses of parents with developmentally disabled children will be discussed. Roles and interactions of family members, particularly those of parents, single parents, and siblings, will also be discussed. Crisis situations that the family encounters during adolescence will be reviewed. Finally, the family's use of support services will be discussed.

## THE FAMILY

There are many reasons for considering the family as the unit of service. According to Ruth Freeman (1970) the family is the "natural and fundamental" unit of society. The long duration of the family experience, which exists in some form throughout the world and includes virtually every individual, the intimacy of the contacts, and the social and legal obligations imposed by family membership, make the family an institution that involves the majority of the population. The level of general family functioning, the degree to which the family can move as a unit to deal with its problems and to maximize the function of the potential of each of its members, will profoundly influence health matters. Consequently the quality of family functioning is of central concern to the nurse working with the developmentally disabled adolescent.

## PARENTING ROLE

Being a parent is an all encompassing role. Helen Perlman (1970) described the parenting role as a consuming, emotionally invested one. It involves a person's deepest feelings and fullest powers of understanding and planning. Parenting requires interaction with the other parent, each child in the family, and the children as a group. It also necessitates involvement outside the immediate family with societal expectations and cultural norms that are generally well defined for the "normal" child but that remain ill-defined for the child who varies from the norm.

### The Meaning of a Child to the Parents

Our culture thinks of the birth of a baby as one of the most exciting events in life. The very idea of creating a new person is awesome. According to Howell (1973), parents enjoy the thought of reproducing themselves by giving birth to a healthy beautiful child. They seek self-fulfillment and hope to become fuller human beings through their child. This fulfillment is not experienced with the birth of a handicapped child. Producing such offspring is especially painful when the culture involved, like the American culture, places high importance on success, beauty, and perfection. Consequently, when parents learn that their child has one or more handicaps they experience disappointment, frustration, and sorrow over the loss of their perfect child, instead of the anticipated joy and excitement.

Wounded pride and feelings of guilt may predominate over the expected joy and caring. This can result in rejection of the child. Aside from dealing with their grief, parents must adjust to their handicapped child. First, when parents have just learned about the handicap they may be in a state of disintegration, shock or emotional numbness. Next, they may become irrational, deny, or search for a magical cure. The third stage is called reintegration and is reached when parents have been able to cope successfully (Howell, 1973).

## Parental Responses

Families' reactions in learning to live with their handicapped child are recognizable though they may vary, depending on the expectations of the child and of the parenting role, the sociocultural and religious orientation, and individual emotional strengths and weaknesses.

Simon Olshansky (1962) has hypothesized that most parents have a pervasive psychological reaction of chronic sorrow throughout their lives, whether the child is at home or not. There may be variations at different times in different situations for different families. Some parents may be able to express their sorrow more openly than others.

Olshansky submits that what is often viewed as denial of the condition is really denial of the chronic sorrow that parents are showing. Professionals may have a tendency to view it as denial of the handicapping condition since expression of sorrow is more difficult to deal with and may be viewed as neurotic, rather than as a natural and understandable response to a tragic fact.

Guilt, shame, anger, and depression are also related to the grief. After the initial shock and initial denial, during the process of recognition, feelings of guilt often arise out of feeling disappointment and personal inadequacy.

Ambivalence toward the child and anger toward others who do not have this fate are also expected reactions. As parents generally find it difficult to allow themselves to recognize and to express this anger, depression ensues. As some of these feelings are resolved, the parents become freer to recognize the problems and to accept the "difference." They are then able to begin to mobilize their efforts and achieve some reintegration, gathering their resources.

Even though parents may be able to find relatively good resolution to the above mentioned stresses, more intense feelings and reactions arise again at points of crises in their and their child's lives, such as adolescence.

Viewed comparatively, the stresses of living with or having a developmentally disabled child are much greater than those experienced with "normal" children. Olshansky points out that, while parents of normal children endure many woes, trials, and moments of despair, they know that eventually the child will be a self-sufficient adult. With the disabled child, there is the anticipation that there will be constant demands and constant dependency, and the knowledge that all woes are going to continue until one's own or the child's death. Thus, parental reactions to disabled children are not necessarily different from reactions to other children, but they are more intense and more prolonged. The excessive and long standing dependency burdens are emotionally draining.

## The Parents and the Adolescent

With many developmentally disabled children, a pattern of overprotectiveness is often established between the parents and the youngster. This is often the parents' way of protecting themselves, even more than their child, from the hurt that they experience in relating to the world around them. With approaching adolescence, the interdependence between parents and child is threatened. The mother who generally has had more intensive involvement on a daily or hourly basis with the child may overprotect the adolescent. The thought of exposing oneself and one's child to the world becomes a threat, as the following case study of Miss M. and her family illustrates.

Miss M., a severely disabled youngster, has a family, who, by their overprotection, have made her adjustment to the outside world even more difficult than it would otherwise need to have been. Miss M. was brought to an interdisciplinary child development center for a full evaluation at age 13. She was a severely physically disabled cerebral palsied child who demonstrated potential for intellectual growth. She had been cared for almost exclusively by her family—mother, father, and several siblings—with no appropriate schooling in the various parts of the world where the family had lived. The family claimed that every time they were ready to have evaluation and treatment they had to move. Although Miss M. had no muscle control and no speech, the family worked out a refined communication system, with mother being the main "interpreter" for the child. The mother's needs for seeing herself as an adequate mother were being met through the interdependent, almost symbiotic relationship with Miss M. Despite the basically sound acceptance of Miss M. in the family and the warmth and caring surrounding this child, there were elements of overprotection. Over the years, the family had sought minimal medical and educational attention. Developing a communication system that could not be transferred to relationships with people outside the family, rather than seeking aid to obtain appropriate training, was another way of overprotecting the child and denying her the opportunity to develop her very limited potential for communication. Managing to never quite complete evaluation allowed the family to protect themselves from the hurt of having all their fears of the nonreversibility of Miss M.'s condition confirmed.

As Miss M. and her family completed a thorough evaluation process involving ten disciplines at the child development center, detailed recommendations were made which included developing Miss M.'s limited motor skills to permit her to use mechanical aids such as a communication board. Although the family had indicated that they wanted such help, there was a great deal of resistance to beginning consistent use of these aids. The family had an investment in keeping Miss M. the helpless child whose needs had to be met totally by others in the family in order to validate their self-concept as the good mother and mother substitute, and to sublimate their feelings of anger and guilt. Siblings were also drawn into the interdependence, relating to the child in an almost "like a mother" manner. Fostering total dependency upon family members results only in making a possible future need to adjust to another living situation a very difficult transition for the disabled person. The mother, or others in the family who are in such an interdependent relationship with the disabled person, may experience emotional difficulty when the need for separation occurs.

Parents who have been overinvested in the child may find it increasingly difficult to use available support systems, such as the extended family, educational and community resources, or health care intervention. They may have cut off even those supports that are clearly available and even mandatory for their child. Stigma becomes another source of strain for such parents, which keeps to a minimum the interaction between the disabled child with anyone beyond the immediate family. This might put the home in isolation and would certainly tend to isolate the mother (Carver, 1972). The parents' ability to benefit from the support systems depends on their own strengths and their acceptance of reality. If parents have been able to use available support systems, or develop their own, by the time their child has become an adolescent he will have had an opportunity to observe and emulate models for relating to people outside the family. There might thus be a better chance for him to optimize his social relationship potential and to begin to build his own support systems.

## FAMILY PROBLEMS

Studies have shown that families of the developmentally disabled, and the mentally retarded particularly, often have more problems than other families in individual and marital adjustment, child rearing practices, and sibling relationships. They are significantly affected socially, economically, and emotionally, and the impact is on all members of the family unit (Schild, 1976). Difficulties in patterns of relating among other family members become intensified and more primitive aspects of family relationships re-emerge. Unresolved issues with the parents' own emancipation may arise, and unhappiness about the parents' marriage may be displaced onto the child.

### The Child Living with One Parent

Developmentally disabled individuals living in one-parent families may have additional difficulties in coping. In relation to the prevalence of one parent families among handicapped children, the potential for separation and divorce is higher among families having a developmentally disabled child. The stress of a damaged self-image is considered as contributing to the need for a particularly vulnerable parent to separate himself or herself from the family situation. On the other hand, there may be increased anger and guilt about leaving the handicapped individual with the other parent. If parents remain together "because of the child" it is even more likely than in other situations with the handicapped that the child will become a displaced focal point of family stress, and consequently, his development and care may be further hampered. If parents separate, with one parent's difficulty in acceptance of the handicapped child as the alleged precipitating factor, it is unlikely that the child would be able to have as positive a relationship with the parent who is not in his household as he would if the separation had had another precipitating factor. In addition, the disabled child would have more difficulty accepting the parent leaving the household than would his siblings, even if this were well interpreted to him. Thus, when parents have marital difficulty, the developmentally disabled individual's growth may be hampered more than his siblings', whether or not his parents remain together. Living in a household with two parents who are too guilt-ridden to separate may also place additional burdens of confusion, hostility and unexplained feelings on the handicapped individual. If parents separate or one parent dies, siblings may be drawn into even further unwarranted taking of responsibility.

A loss of a parent by death, an extremely traumatic event in any young person's life, takes on much greater proportions for the developmentally disabled child, with the possibility of arrest and regression in development.

## Adolescence as a Family Crisis Period

When equilibrium is disturbed by stressful situations or periods, families make an attempt to adapt to the new situation by using the resources available to them from within the family, as well as from the environment. With a family that is raising a developmentally disabled young person there are times which represent particularly difficult crisis points. The shock at birth is usually the initial crisis. At the time of school entrance parents are forced to observe their child in relation to the environment, and it becomes more difficult to maintain the pretense that "everything will be all right." More exposure to peers hurts parents, as here, too, they witness differences and possible rejection.

Adolescence is also a significant period of crisis. Vocational planning, training, and adjustment become a new and difficult reality. The "normal" child has had certain opportunities for considering vocational possibilities—play, peers, school and camp experiences, and part-time jobs. This may not always be the case for the developmentally disabled. The handicapped young person may have lacked these experiences and may, therefore, have unrealistic fantasies or limited ability to test reality. He may deny his limitations or he may choose to remain in the security of the feeling that he cannot do many things and assesses himself too pessimistically.

At times of general family crisis, such as births, deaths, and shifts in family constellation by marriage, the family is confronted with major decisions, and the need for ongoing care of the disabled individual may again come to the forefront. This is particularly difficult for overinvolved parents, as they are confronted with the interdependence existing between them and their offspring.

Crisis points are particularly advantageous times for the family to take advantage of professional intervention. If a family learns to use its strengths in problem solving, it can attain a better level of functioning after the crisis than it had before.

## THE SIBLING ROLE

The role of siblings is to provide objects for identification and differentiation on a peer level. Distinctive features of sibling relationships are: 1) their inclusive character, 2) the extensiveness of their contacts, and 3) the frankness of the relationships. Children living in the same family act as teachers to one another and they give each other a sense of security (Adamovics, 1960). When a developmentally disabled child is involved, the siblings' role in providing opportunities for testing, establishing and defining competitive strivings, and providing an object for identification and differentiation is still present, but the disabled child is not capable of responding in the "normal" or expected way.

It has been found in some studies (Adamovics, 1960), that when mothers spend more time in care for and in leisure time activities with the disabled child, the siblings experience this as stress which in some cases may constitute maternal deprivation. If the father's attention to the disabled child and to the siblings is more equally divided, then paternal attention may sometimes serve as a compensatory device for lack of maternal attention to either the siblings or the disabled child.

When the developmentally disabled individual is mentally retarded he always remains in the youngest child role in the family. If he is chronologically older, he changes gradually to the youngest child's role. The disabled child who is not mentally retarded but physically handicapped may often continue to need the specialized care that keeps him in a role of getting the attention required as a younger child, while attempting to help him shift to the role of an older sibling in terms of chronological, mental, and emotional growth. Positive opportunities for caring and empathy toward the developmentally disabled individual can exist for the siblings if parents are able to be supportive of such efforts. Parents and other adults in the family need to constantly recognize the needs of all the children in the family. This is particularly important during adolescence.

If the siblings feel left out of parental attention, they may chose various mechanisms for gaining attention. Somatic complaints or acting out behavior of various kinds may be used (Schild, 1976). The burden of parental expectations of ongoing care of the disabled siblings in adult years may alienate the other children from the parents and draw them into an intense anger-guilt struggle. As the siblings approach adolescence and young adulthood, they may also experience fear in relation to marriage and having children even in those cases where this fear is known to be unfounded. Consequently, it is important to include siblings in various aspects of the family's health care in relation to the disabled individual.

In general, there seems to be an interrelationship among the factors related to the developmentally disabled individual's interpretation to the family and acceptance in it. The better the parents themselves are able to understand and accept the disabled individual, the better they can cope with the necessity of interpreting him to the other children in the family. This in turn affects their understanding and acceptance of the child. Furthermore, the more siblings understand and accept their handicapped sibling, the better they are able to explain the child to their friends and to cope with their friends' reactions. Basically this succession of interrelated factors depends upon family solidarity and upon the parents' strengths in coping with a developmentally disabled child in their family.

Having and living with a developmentally disabled brother or sister does not have to be an adverse experience for other children in the family. In fact, it can provide additional dimensions of family solidarity with extra opportunities for developing traits of empathy, caring, and unselfishness. This is possible if the adult members of the family are emotionally free to help create a positive atmosphere to foster such traits in all family members.

## SERVICES

The developmental disability of an individual is a many faceted problem that the family is not able to handle alone. Families struggling to cope with this problem ". . . need equally appropriate and available services, as do families wrestling with other social problems, such as economic difficulties, mental illness, and delinquency. Whenever the stresses of a difficult life situation threaten the intactness and mental health of the family, interventive services may often strategically assist families to attain healthier resolutions to the social problem" (Schild, 1976).

### Basic Needs

Families may need assistance in problem solving that is not specifically related to diagnosis or care of the disabled child. When a family is experiencing the stress of dealing with a disability in one of its members, both the energy spent dealing with the disability and the stigma attached to disability generally in our society make meeting the basic needs of the total family more difficult. Thus, families may have severe problems in relation to meeting the family's need for adequate housing, nutrition, education, employment, and basic health care. Moreover, until such needs are met, the family is not likely to concentrate on dealing fully with the disability. Thus, there should be an opportunity for assistance in meeting basic needs, as part of helping the family gather its strengths to cope with the adversity of the developmentally disabled child.

## Family Service Needs

Until relatively recently, the trend in the health care professions was toward specialization. Thus, each aspect of a medical condition was being treated by a different professional. This resulted in fragmentation and inadequate service and the tendency for parents to "shop around." It may be, however, that the "seeking for the answer they want to hear" was encouraged by the lack of coordination of services and by the professionals' own difficulties in dealing with disability. Certainly it was inadequate from the point of view of involving the patient and the patient's family in the treatment process in such a manner that would enable them to feel that they were members of the team, and decision makers in charge of their own fate. During the last decade, and especially in the last 5 years, there have been attempts to make significant changes in the area of interdisciplinary training, which is slowly beginning to have an impact on the service delivery system and well coordinated family centered care.

The increasing knowledge of each other's expertise by members of the various professions comprising the health care team, and the increasing comfort of these professionals in truly working together in dealing with the total human being and the total family unit within the context of its community, is making it easier for families to relate to the services and to feel part of the team. It is also assuring for families to have continuity of care over the years by one facility, forming alliance with the institution and not only with individual professionals in it.

The professional responsibility for giving clear, precise information to the parents has only recently been given attention in the literature. Matheny and Vernick (1968) hold the view that ". . . what the parents require most from diagnostic or informative counseling is specific, clearly transmitted, honest information about the child, implications for his future, and knowledge of what concrete steps they can take to deal with the problem."

It is important to recognize that the facts of the child's condition have to be clearly presented with a constant testing of whether or not they have been understood. However, if parents have not had an opportunity to work through their expected emotional reactions to the disability, they may not be in a position to hear even the most clearly presented statement.

## Strategy

The more there has been an opportunity to help parents deal with their reactions and the more they can feel part of the professional team in a decision-making capacity, the more likely it will be that effective planning for the affected individual can take place. Thus, it is important to help parents gain enough emotional freedom to be able to hear information and recommendations about their child, to consider them for acceptance, and eventually choose to implement or not to implement them. Hopefully, parents can plan for their adolescent in a responsible manner, with repeated opportunities to reintegrate this information and to reassess the shifts in their adolescent's and their own situation with professional help.

Plans for major changes in the developmentally disabled child's living situation require high adaptive skills both for the adolescent and for the parents. For example, in planning residential institutional placement for a young adolescent, a short term experience with temporary placement can be of help in preparing for future placement. The professional attention received at that time is of great carryover value to the families. Curry (1974) describes the handling of one such plan of respite care leading to future placement:

> The separation anxiety and traumatic impact of placement can be alleviated or minimized by a professional nurse who intervenes to assist the family in preparing for the experience, coordinates the care provided for the child and serves as liaison between the family and child during placement.

The nurse, in other words, may be able to give the parents emotional support, encouragement, practical guidance and suggestions. In residential settings in general the nurse and other members of the nursing staff have a particularly important role in helping the parents relate to the realities of their child's life, to his problem areas and to his successes.

Thus, brief periods of "trying on" a new plan with interpretive and supportive help during these periods can have beneficial effects for instituting the plan on a long term basis and for carry-over to provide less anxious transitory periods of being at home. Seeing the institution in operation and being able to talk about it openly also gives the family a free choice to accept it or reject it.

## Referrals to Mental Health Professionals

Many parents, as well as the developmentally disabled individuals themselves, need an opportunity to work with a mental health professional in a preventive, integrative, or therapeutic way at various times throughout their life. If the work with the mental health professional has been a good experience, possibly at the time of a crisis, parents are more likely to seek such help again. The need to do so should not be viewed as regression or indication of emotional ill health. Some health care professionals occasionally hesitate to refer parents of the developmentally disabled to other health care professionals—to psychiatric nurses, social workers, psychologists, psychiatrists. If any health care worker becomes aware of parental or family indications of turmoil, uncertainties, fears, anger, or depression, and chooses not to relate to this by direct intervention or referral, a disservice is done to the family. The message to the family then is, "We don't talk about this here," or "It is not O.K. to have those feelings." Thus, the parents' guilt is reinforced. If attention is not given to the emotional aspects of the disability and to their implications for the family, the family may not be able to integrate or use nearly as well the practical planning and programming for the child. There is an interrelationship between these, as noted earlier. As parents become more free and open with their emotions, they can use concrete suggestions for planning better. Once there is an increased ease with the care of the handicapped individual in their daily life, parents may become more able to deal with their own emotional needs.

## Family Centered Services

A wide variety of services is needed to help sustain the developmentally disabled young person and his family. Service needs magnify as the young person reaches adolescence and young adulthood. These needs and how they are being met by community facilities—vocational, medical and social—are described in other chapters in this book. Family needs that have to be met at least partly by professional intervention outside the family, include: 1) internal conflicts that are reactivated by stress, particularly around crisis points occurring at adolescence, 2) concerns about family functioning, including siblings and members of the extended family, 3) guidance around the developmental stages blurred by the handicap, 4) information about the handicap and treatment programs, 5) interpretation of community resources, and 6) counseling for siblings, including genetic counseling, where indicated.

## PROFESSIONAL APPROACHES

The skills needed in working with families of the developmentally disabled are the same as working with other families. These include sensitivity to the parents' problems, helping them express their feelings, offering and interpreting the agency's services constructively, examining with the family the choices available in dealing with their problem, and sustaining them in the choice they make.

Many different professionals intervene with a developmentally disabled individual. The role of nursing personnel spreads over various levels of intervention. Prevention, recognition, referral, and ongoing direct patient care in the home and in institutions, as well as involvement with public and private health care systems, are all areas where nurses function. Since in health care settings the nurse spends more time with the patient than does any other member of the team, she is in the unique position of observing interaction between the patient and members of the family on a consistent and frequent basis. She has the advantage of being able to intervene therapeutically in a timely fashion. The nurse can also be a primary caregiver, researcher, and consultant to other disciplines.

Preventive and therapeutic intervention with adolescents and families in relation to their mental health needs can take the form of individual, couples, or family therapy; individual child therapy; and group therapy with parents, siblings, or multiple families. The appropriate combination of treatment services is based on a sensitive and thorough diagnostic understanding of the family.

An important support system for parents is provided by other parents. The common bonds among parents of the developmentally disabled have been one of the cornerstones for building the effective parent organizations and subsequent "parent power" which has been instrumental in achieving progress in legislation, services, and generally better acceptance of developmental disabilities. The involvement of parents, professionals, and the public in this growing advocacy movement is described in more detail elsewhere in this book.

Parenting with a developmentally disabled child is at best a most demanding task, requiring unexpected role adaptations. The degree to which parents make these adaptations depends on their ability to use their inner resources, to build supports and to avail themselves of existing support systems in the context of their extended family and community.

## Professional Self-Awareness

Although we as professionals may feel grief in seeing a handicapped child, it is important to allow ourselves to feel this sadness, and to recognize the intensity of our own reactions. As we learn to accept our own feelings, we can become increasingly effective in our own work on behalf of the developmentally disabled and their families. Some of us may experience guilt about feeling relieved because we do not have that particular misfortune in our life. If we are not aware of this, we cannot deal constructively with the parents' anger and frustration.

## CONCLUSION

Many families show great strength in establishing and maintaining equilibrium in their family. They are able to integrate their lives and their children's lives to meet the needs of the total family. Parental responses to a handicapped individual should be considered by all who work with families who have a developmentally disabled child. Adolescence can be a crisis period to the family as well as to the teenager himself. Single parents and their handicapped children have special needs, as do siblings. There are a number of considerations to be made in planning family centered care during the adolescent period. Finally, professionals need to be aware of their own feelings and responses to handicapped individuals and their families.

## REFERENCES CITED

Adamovics, I. 1960. Siblings' responses to the mentally retarded child's presence in the family. In: I. Adamovics, Frei F., Legaré P., McIntosh D., and Rubin P. The Impact of the Mentally Retarded Child on the Family Unit, pp. 233–313. Unpublished M.S.W. group thesis. McGill University School of Social Work.

Carver, J., and Carver, N. E. 1972. The Family of the Retarded Child. Syracuse University Press, Syracuse.

Curry, J. B. 1974. Nursing intervention during temporary care. Ment. Retard. 12:1:17–19.

Freeman, R. 1970. Community Health Nursing. W. B. Saunders, Philadelphia.

Hill, R. 1968. Generic features of families under stress. Soc. Casework 39(2-3):139–150.

Howell, S. E. 1973. Psychiatric aspects of habilitation. Pediatr. Clin. N. Am. 20(1):203–219.

Matheny, A. P., Jr., and Vernick, J. 1968. Parents of the mentally retarded child: Emotionally overwhelmed or informationally deprived? J. Pediatr. 74:953–959.

Olshansky, S. 1962. Chronic sorrow: A response to having a mentally defective child. Soc. Casework 43:191–194.

Perlman, H. H. 1970. Help to parents of the mentally retarded child: Diagnostic focus. In: M. Schreiber, Social Work and Mental Retardation, pp. 346–356. The John Day Co., New York.

Schild, S. 1976. The family of the retarded child. In: R. Koch and J. C. Dobson (eds.), The Mentally Retarded Child and the Family—A Multidisciplinary Handbook. Brunner-Mazel, New York.

## Suggested Readings

Aguilcra, D. C., Messick, J. M. and Farrell, M. 1974. Crisis Intervention: Theory and Methodology. C. V. Mosby, St. Louis.

Baranyay, E. P. 1971. The Mentally Handicapped Adolescent Pergamon Press, Oxford.

Begab, M. J., and Richardson, S. A. (eds.). 1975. The Mentally Retarded and Society—A Social Science Perspective. University Park Press, Baltimore.

Dempsey, J. J. (ed.). 1975. Community Services for Retarded Children: The Consumer-Provider Relationship. University Park Press, Baltimore.

Farber, B. 1960. Family organization and crisis: Maintenance of integration in families with a severely mentally retarded child. Monogr. Soc. Res. Child Dev. 25(75):1.

Farber, B. 1968. Mental Retardation—Its Social Context and Social Consequences. Houghton, Mifflin, Boston.

Marshall, A. H., Jr. 1973. An investigation into the perceptions of interpersonal communication of educable mentally retarded adolescents and their mothers. Diss. Abstr. 34A(9):5757–5758.

Mercer, R. Th. 1974. Responses of five multigravidae to the event of the birth of an infant with a defect. Diss. Abstr. 34B(10):5040–5041.

Mesibov, G. R. 1976. Alternatives to the principle of normalization. Ment. Retard. 14(5):30–32.

Michaelis, C. G. 1974. Chip on my shoulder. Except. Parent. 4(1):30–35.

Miller, S. G. 1974. An exploratory study of sibling relationships in families with retarded children. Diss. Abstr. 35B(6):2994–2995.

Noland, R. L. (ed.). 1970. Counseling Parents of the Mentally Retarded—A Sourcebook. Charles C Thomas, Springfield, Ill.

Rapoport, L. 1965. The State of Crisis: Some theoretical considerations. In: H. Parad, Crisis Intervention: Selected Readings, Family Service Association, New York, 368 p.

Robinson, L. H. 1974. Group work with parents of retarded adolescents. Am. J. of Psychother. 18(3):397–408.

Schreiber, M. 1970. Social Work and Mental Retardation. The John Day Co., New York.

Segal, R. M. 1970. Mental Retardation and Social Action. Charles C Thomas, Springfield, Ill.

Throne, J. M. 1975. Normalization through the normalization principle: right ends, wrong means. Ment. Retard. 13(5):23–25.

Veeder, N. W. 1974. A stress-strength model for nurse-social worker collaboration. Ment. Retard. 12(2):39–42.

Wolfensberger, W. 1972. Normalization—The Principle of Normalization in Human Services. National Institute of Mental Retardation, Toronto.

Wolff, I. 1964. Nursing Role in Counseling Parents of Mentally Retarded Children. U.S. Dept. of Health, Education, and Welfare, Welfare Administration, Children's Bureau, Washington, D.C.

# chapter six

# THE ADOLESCENT IN THE COMMUNITY

Virginia Williams, M.A.

For generations, the primary concept of residential service for the developmentally disabled has been terminal placement in an institution. Professionals, beginning with the family doctor and clergy, would frequently advise parents that their developmentally disabled child be separated from family and community—"for the good of everyone concerned." Most parents, even when they wanted desperately to keep their child at home, were faced with the realization that limited supportive services were available (Krause, 1976). Historically, the developmentally disabled have been denied not only a free and appropriate education, but they have had little protection against abuses as a result of inadequate care and education. More recently, there has been a significant trend toward deinstitutionalization and development of community-based residential facilities and services for developmentally disabled individuals, a national movement which constitutes one of this century's most dramatic trends in human services.

Progressive state governments have begun to change their traditional custodial role by initiating innovative programs that prepare residents for the transition to community placement. For example, in the state of Pennsylvania some 2,000 persons with developmental disabilities, in a four year period, were placed in community-based facilities. Satellite agencies and regional centers have appeared on the community scene. Supportive services, based in the community, have increased. Transition from institution to the community has become a reality for more (Krause, 1976). This chapter discusses residential living alternatives and the community service needs of the developmentally disabled adolescent. It also reviews obstacles to community service delivery for the developmentally disabled. The deinstitutionalization process is reviewed as well as the role that institutional personnel should play in that process. Finally, the need for community education is reviewed.

## RESIDENTIAL LIVING ALTERNATIVES

There is now demonstrable evidence that the developmentally disabled can live successfully in the community in several types of residential alternatives to institutions. These include their own homes, foster homes, small group homes, apartments, and independent community residential settings. The availability of well developed community residential services provides the key to effective normalization, mainstreaming, and deinstitutionalization. Provided with training and guidance, a large majority of people in these alternative residences are earning their livings and the respect of their neighbors as well (Krause, 1976). Residential alternatives have the potential of providing the developmentally disabled individual and his family with a series of options—options essential to the continued development of the entire family. The learning environment is expanded, the limits on opportunity are dramatically reduced and the community's resources are more appropriately used. The economic gains to the community have been documented, both in terms of human resources and costs of operation. By comparing the costs for life, time, and services for the mentally retarded, in Table 1 further illustrates this point.

A service system based upon individual need does not demand that an individual accept services that he does not require (Cherington and Dywadie, 1974). For example, not all developmentally disabled require a residential service. Those who do need supervised living arrangements, do not all need the same type of residential service. In order to make the service system economic as well as humane, it is essential that a variety of options be available to fit the individual requirements of the developmentally disabled individual throughout his life as is illustrated in Figure 1.

## DEINSTITUTIONALIZATION

To follow an adolescent through the deinstitutionalization process there are many steps to be considered.

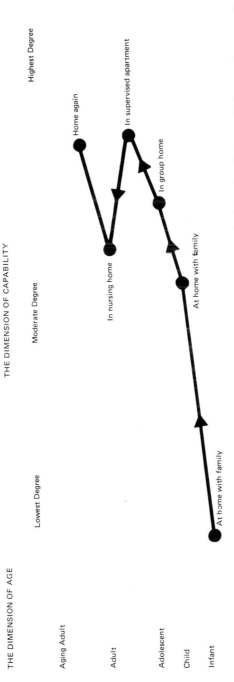

Figure 1.  Hypothetical case of an individual's need for shelter. Movement of the line indicates the dimension of change which occurs in a person's need for shelter as he develops and ages. The dimensions of individuality and of choice are highlighted by critical decision points (marked by arrows). From: Cherington and Dywadie (eds.), *New Neighbors: The Retarded Citizen in Quest of a Home*, 1974. President's Committee on Mental Retardation, Washington, D.C.

Table 1. Comparison of costs for lifetime services[a]

| | |
|---|---:|
| Placed in institution at age 6 for lifetime (till 65 @ $5,252 per year) | $309,868 |
| Placed in institution for lifetime (till 65 @ $12,118 per year) | 714,962 |
| (Based on per diem costs FY 70) | |
| Mildly retarded lives at home, becomes independent | |
|   Preschool 2 years ($1,000 per year) | 2,000 |
|   School 5–18, EMR ($700 per year) | 9,100 |
|   Transitional workshop, 18 mos ($1,600 per year) | 2,400 |
| | $ 13,500 |
| | |
| Mildly retarded without suitable homes, in small group homes | |
|   Community services | $ 13,500 |
|   Boarding home, 6–16 ($2,500 per year) | 25,000 |
|              16–18 ($1,700 per year) | 3,400 |
|   Hostel, 18–20 ($1,700 per year) | 3,400 |
| | $ 45,300 |
| | |
| Moderately retarded with home, community services | |
|   Preschool day training, 4–6 ($1,600 per year) | $ 3,200 |
|   TMR class, 6–19 ($1,200 per year) | 15,600 |
|   Sheltered workshop and extended employment, 20–26, ($1,300 per year) | 58,500 |
| | 77,300 |
|   Group homes, 6–65 ($2,500 per year) | 75,000 |
| | $152,300 |

Moderately retarded without suitable home
Community services .................................................................................. $ 77,300
Group home, 6–65 ($2,500 per year) ............................................................ 147,500
$224,800

Severely retarded at home
Day training and work activity, 4–65 ($1,600 per year) ................................. $ 97,600
Group home, 35–65 ($2,500 per year) ......................................................... 75,000
$172,600

Severely retarded in community
Community services .................................................................................. $ 97,600
Group home, 6–65 ($2,500 per year) ............................................................ 147,500
$245,100

ᵃ Taken from *Residential Study: The Georgia and Atlanta Associations for Retarded Children.* January, 1972. Atlanta Association for Retarded Citizens.

## The Identification Process

How is the developmentally disabled adolescent identified as being a potential participant in a habilitative program that prepares him for community living and/or a community program? This identification process should be done by institution personnel with the help and guidance of the local Department of Vocational Rehabilitation and other community agencies responsible for the continued comprehensive care and service to the adolescent. This may vary according to locale. In some locations the responsible agency might be the Department of Welfare. Whatever screening and evaluation and habilitation program is established for the developmentally disabled adolescent, if done in conjunction with the community agency involved, it will be more supportive to the individual.

## The Transition Process

Once it is determined by the appropriate "screening teams" that the adolescent is ready for the transition, another person or persons joins the team. For the individual leaving the institution in order to reside in a group home, the counselor from the group home becomes a member of the team.

## Job Placement

The adolescent may, after training, be placed in a job. It is not the responsibility of the employer to become the counselor or guardian to his recently employed developmentally disabled adolescent. The person identified in the community agency and the counselors of the group home must become job counselors. They should remain in touch with the employer and ward off the possibility of having the adolescent fired after a brief period of work. Job placement is probably one of the most difficult steps. Consequently, job expectations must be a part of the habilitative and training program. An interdisciplinary team for the employee should be consulted prior to employment.

## Community Program

If space has been found for the adolescent to participate in a sheltered workshop program the transition is sometimes easier. Staff members in a sheltered workshop provide programs that allow the adolescent to adjust to community living. The sheltered workshop can provide on-site employment as well as job training for employment in the community.

## Support Services

Whatever the living arrangements for the developmentally disabled adolescent, support services must be readily available. Such services include an individualized program plan with:

1. income security
2. transportation
3. educational
4. health care
5. vocational alternatives
6. recreation
7. parent support
8. advocacy
9. on going placement evaluation (Braddock, 1976)

## COMMUNITY SERVICE NEEDS OF THE DEVELOPMENTALLY DISABLED

There needs to be a diversity of community services available to the developmentally disabled adolescent. These services should be provided by local community agencies. These services must include those listed above. In addition, appropriate services and support systems need to be available for caretakers of the developmentally disabled in the community, particularly for natural families of severely handicapped individuals. The provision of respite care offers the family relief in the care of their child and subsequently lessens strain on the family unit. Every family needs some privacy and quiet time. With a severely handicapped child or adult at home, such opportunities are often minimal. Placing the handicapped individual in a temporary foster home, residential camp program, or a residential care facility during a weekend, family vacation, or in terms of acute stress, can provide the needed break allowing family members to renew their outlook in dealing with the problems of the developmentally disabled (Thompson, 1976).

## OBSTACLES TO COMMUNITY SERVICE DELIVERY

Community agencies face many problems in their attempt to provide needed services to the developmentally disabled adolescent. Because of their diversity, the needs of the developmentally disabled adolescent cut across the services of many community agencies. Most agencies are unfamiliar and uncomfortable with this group, preferring to work with the nonhandicapped population whom they feel they understand. Such agencies are often caught in budgetary and funding difficulties. By having to deliver services to yet another group they may feel a new burden. Service and staff costs, which are often unpredictable, further complicate the process of seeking funds. Lack of cooperation and support between agencies often occurs. The net result is denial of community service by one agency if a second agency needs to be involved. For example, an adolescent who is labeled mentally retarded, but who also has a hearing impairment, may not receive the attention of the agency providing speech and hearing services because he has been classified as retarded. A cerebral palsied adolescent who is not mentally retarded may be placed in a special education program regardless of whether or not it is needed. Ultimately, the most successful community programs for the developmentally disabled adolescent are those that provide health services, education, vocational rehabilitation, welfare, and social services. All of these agencies have the potential for the development of programs within the community for the adolescent who is developmentally disabled.

## INTERAGENCY COMMUNICATION

In order for existing community agencies to establish community alternatives for the developmentally disabled there must be a system of interagency communication. Interagency communication cannot be mandated. You must:

1. determine the limitation of agencies—what services they can provide and to whom
2. discover if there is an overlap of services provided by different agencies
3. find out what is the legislative mandate to the agency

If a developmentally disabled adolescent needs the services of the Department of Vocational Rehabilitation and the local social services agency to provide a complete service and rehabilitative program, then these two agencies, once aware of the needs of the adolescent, should work together to provide the full service base needed to maintain the developmentally disabled adolescent in the community. Again, it is important that we remember not to ask an agency to provide a service they do not have the expertise to provide, or to cross boundaries and infringe on another agency. It is our responsibility to assure one agency that where their services end, another agency is available to "pick up" the other end and continue the provision of services.

## THE ROLE OF THE INSTITUTION STAFF

Institution staff should play a major role in the deinstitutionalization process. Unfortunately, among people working in the institution, deinstitutionalization has often meant the loss of a job. Deinstitutionalization has also meant an economic loss to the community where the institution is located and, consequently, resistance to alternative placements for the developmentally disabled has developed. One solution to this dilemma is to develop skills among institutional personnel which will enable them to make the transition from institution to community employment with the developmentally disabled population. Recently, some colleges and universities have been involved in establishing training programs for institution staff. An example of such a program was conducted by George Washington University and Forest Haven, a public institution in Laurel, Maryland, for the retarded residents of the District of Columbia. Through a grant provided by the Department of Health, Education, and Welfare, a life skills program was established at Forest Haven. The major focus was the training of institution staff to assess the needs of community residents and implement a life skills program. The University Affiliated Program for Child Development at Georgetown University Hospital has also been actively involved in training such institution staff at Forest Haven. The purpose of the training has been to teach staff how to assess the institutionalized population in order to determine the level of functioning of the individuals and the type of individual program necessary to begin to prepare the individual for some community alternatives.

This training has, for the most part, been geared to enhance the skills of counselors, teachers, health aides, and all who work directly with the individual in the institution. Training programs such as these should be developed to help build additional skills among institutional staff. Such training will help them make a successful transition to new careers in the community. The institution staff could thus play a major role in assisting the developmentally disabled individual in maintaining himself in the community. With additional training, counselors, teachers, and health aides could be expected to assume new roles and responsibilities such as teaching the developmentally disabled individual to travel independently, by initially accompanying the developmentally disabled individual. The developmentally disabled individual, whether living in a group home, in a day care facility, in a foster home, or more independently in an apartment, will need training in many areas that institutional living did not require. Staff from institutions should also be encouraged to become advocates for the people they have been serving within the institution. An advocacy group to assure alternative placement for the developmentally disabled adolescent is essential in the continuum of care for this population. Such a group could also talk to small neighborhood groups, to local PTA's, and to parent groups. An additional role that institution personnel could play is to maintain the records that will follow the adolescent into his community placement. Any professional in contact with a developmentally disabled adolescent should be able to depend upon the institution staff to provide information about the individual that will help maintain him in the community.

## COMMUNITY EDUCATION

Community education is necessary to accomplish any of the goals of deinstitutionalization. Communities have fought the establishment of community residences for the developmentally disabled population because of a lack of understanding of the developmentally disabled individual. Local zoning regulations and special land use regulations have blocked the establishment of a community based residence. Through community concern and support changes in these regulations can be made. There are several groups that can initiate programs of community awareness. The first, and possibly one of the most important groups is the clergy. The Red Cross, the Lions Club, and the Kiwanis Club are community groups that can help prepare the community and assist community agencies in developing programs and facilities. Programs or facilities established without the support or at least the awareness of the community will fail. An important factor in a program of community education is to teach the community that the developmentally disabled adolescent is not a purse snatcher, a rapist, or a child molester, but an individual with a disability who has the right to participate in the community.

## CONCLUSION

Change is not easy. When people are faced with new ideas, preconceptions, or prejudices it is often easier to give in to them rather than alter them or bring about an actual social change. Attempting to provide a richer life for the developmentally disabled adolescent requires a tremendous amount of work and perseverance. There are no simple rules for success. Guidelines which will be successful in every community do not exist. Ultimately, the responsibility rests on the nurse and other health care professionals to know the facts of an individual community; to establish goals and priorities; to survey and analyze needs, resources, and power structures; and to work with the community and the developmentally disabled individual to plan where and how the developmentally disabled should live in a particular area (NARC, 1973).

## REFERENCES CITED

Braddock, D. 1976. Opening Closed Doors: The Deinstitutionalization of Disabled Individuals. The Council for Exceptional Children. Reston, Va.

Cherington, and Dywadie. (eds.) 1974. New Neighbors: The Retarded Citizen in Quest of a Home. President's Committee on Mental Retardation. DHEW publication No. (OHD) 74-21004.

Krause, F. J. 1976. Foreword to, People Live in Houses: Profiles of Community Residences for Retarded Children and Adults. President's Committee on Mental Retardation DHEW No. (OMD) 75-21006.

National Association for Retarded Citizens. 1973. The Right to Choose, Achieving Residential Alternatives in the Community. National Association for Retarded Citizens, Arlington, Tex.

Thompson, C. R. 1976. Social work. In: R. J. Johnston and P. R. Magrab (eds.), Developmental Disorders: Assessment, Treatment, Education, pp. 111–127. University Park Press, Baltimore.

# chapter seven
# SPECIAL EDUCATION NEEDS

Michael Bender, Ed.D.

By definition, adolescence can be the best of times and the worst of times. For many individuals it is an age of making decisions for the first time. Traditional definitions of adolescence tend to emphasize chronological age, physical development, and legal restrictions. The adolescent life cycle occurs with a starting age ranging from 10 to 13 and a concluding age varying from 19 to 21 (Lambert et al, 1972). If one defines adolescence in behavioral terms rather than within the limits of traditional parameters it becomes a term which is more workable and meaningful, specifically in light of working with the developmentally disabled.

Adolescence is widely recognized as a developmental period for personal, social, sexual, and, for some, political and religious concerns. Peer adjustment, separation without isolation, and a striving for independence from parents and close family members also characterize this period (Muuss, 1975). For the first time, many adolescents are exposed to pre-work or work situations as well as an abundance of leisure time. It is a time during which guidance systems are being formulated and, for the most part, quickly tested, accepted, or discarded.

It is important to emphasize that every child, handicapped or nonhandicapped, has feelings and experiences pleasure and pain, success or failure, and rejection and acceptance. During the period

This paper was supported in part by the United States Office of Education Grant for Special Education Programs and University Affiliated Facilities (B.E.H.) and by the Joseph P. Kennedy, Jr. Foundation.

defined as adolescence, there is a tendency to overreact to these feelings (Buckler, 1971). The child who is mentally retarded is especially vulnerable to the experiences of rejection or failure. Many of these children have been in school programs which have been nonproductive, and they have learned to accept their lack of achievement and accompanying low esteem as products of their educational programming. As with most adolescents, the developmentally disabled individual acts out his feelings, often disagreeing with, and at times rejecting his parents. This tumultuous period is often characterized by many feelings of personal inadequacy. One unique difficulty experienced by the adolescent who is handicapped and specifically, the mentally retarded adolescent, is that he is often denied the freedom to disagree with parental desires and to break away from close supervision. The child who is not developmentally disabled has many more options available to him in terms of going places, participating in school activities, dating, and interacting in society. Many professionals believe severely developmentally disabled adolescents need to be protected, especially those who exhibit poor judgment, lack of knowledge, and who are susceptible to exploitation or situations which may cause them future problems.

It is interesting to note that, for the mentally retarded, adolescent friendships are often predicted upon rigid standards of what is acceptable to parents rather than on whom the adolescent selects as friends (Dittmann, 1959). It is evident that this population of individuals has many additional problems when compared to the normal adolescent. Mildly retarded adolescents and young adults have continuing special problems which may deter their adjustments, such as lack of self-control and inability to understand the complexities of their environment (Foale, 1956). Many individuals are not only physically handicapped, but may be further handicapped by an inability to reason, to adapt to new situations, and to accept the feelings associated with rejection and failure. Often, developmentally disabled teenagers have been overprotected and lack the social experiences of interacting with their peers or nondevelopmentally disabled individuals. In essence, they are poorly prepared for today's culture and society. Professionals have postulated the view that the adolescent adjustment period for the retarded person may indeed last longer than that anticipated on the basis of mental or chronological age. It is interesting to note that while this has been suggested by many individuals (Saenger, 1957), additional schooling and specialized counseling services which would offer some compensation to these individuals is practically nonexistent.

The importance of peer group associations for the developmentally disabled cannot be overemphasized. Adolescents, finding themselves in transitionary phases moving them toward an increasing level of independence, begin to look to their peers for security and support. Most nonhandicapped adolescents are able to select the peers with whom they form these new alliances and accept or reject peer companionship. An essential aspect of the socialization process for the developmentally disabled must also include informal peer group associations where they can share their attitudes, assess themselves, and select friends (Child, 1953). Countless examples of the need for these associations for the handicapped as well as for the nonhandicapped are documented throughout the literature involving the theories of adolescence. Yet, curricula in most special or regular school programs offer few opportunities for the development of these relationships. Extracurricular activities offer more of an opportunity for these associations to develop (McDaniel, 1970).

It is also important to consider the adjustment problems many developmentally disabled adolescents experience, specifically in regard to their self-concepts. In a study by Collins and Burger (1970) educable mentally retarded adolescents attending special education classes were compared with adolescents attending classes for normal students on the Tennessee Self-Concept Scale. The results supported the view that educably mentally retarded adolescents may very well have a negative self-concept and low self-esteem. Carp (1960) expressed the view that the self-concept of the retarded individual may in part be due to his feelings of being degraded. He suggests that many retarded individuals will become antisocial after being treated unfairly and thus become more firmly rejected by their peers. Barclay and Goulet (1965) suggested that the social maturity of the retarded child may be a result of the degree of acceptance or nonacceptance of the child by his parents and siblings. The confusion as to whether the self-concept of the mentally retarded individual is lower or less developed than that of the normal child is an endless battle. Mayer (1966) supports the view that retarded children do not have negative self-concepts, which runs counter to those who suggest the opposite opinion. The critical question, which is often not addressed by professionals, is how do we enhance the developmentally disabled's self-concept? This specific charge is usually directed to the adolescent's school program, and in many instances is relegated to a minor part of the student's curriculum.

With the start of the adolescent period the family continues to be the main socializing agent, although its authority must be tempered with competing socializing forces such as the adolescents need for independence and peer group associations. For the severely disabled, most of the decisions regarding major changes in living, dating, and even associations are imposed primarily by his parents. Usually the parents seek additional support from outside agencies or the assistance of religious leaders, physicians, nurses or rehabilitation or habilitation agencies. The impact of a developmentally disabled adolescent on a family can indeed be overwhelming. Overprotection by the family may limit the socialization process and may create future problems. Additionally, Farber (1968) has suggested that the chances of being successful in life for most handicapped persons are reduced because these individuals form a part of society which could be considered surplus. Again a cycle is repeated; they are surplus because their chances for being successful in life are so limited. Farber suggests that our social structure with its rigid controls, exacting rules of social organization, and limited number of available positions or openings, penalizes the handicapped individual.

## EDUCATIONAL PROGRAMMING

Educational goals for the developmentally disabled adolescent can vary greatly from those established for students in the regular grades. Many programs for the moderately and severely handicapped have traditionally concentrated upon teaching self-care and socialization skills. Few school programs have offered a comprehensive curriculum which takes into consideration the special needs of the developmentally disabled adolescent. What and how to teach these individuals has long been discussed among educators. Few formal curricula have been developed offering a total program for handicapped students and taking into consideration all levels of disabilities. Curricula developed for the developmentally disabled have tended to ignore or treat lightly vocational and work oriented activities. Development of prevocational skills has often been neglected or given low priority in special education programs. Those skills which teach how to seek employment, how to operate simple equipment and appliances found at home or in the community, or how to be a consumer of goods and services, are often relegated to the student's last year of formal schooling. An added problem is that most public school prevocational or vocational training programs have been concerned primarily with educably retarded students. Those students who have been classified as multiply handicapped or severely and profoundly retarded have traditionally been institutionalized or excluded from formal training programs. An erroneous assumption has been that these students are incapable of intellectually, socially, or emotionally benefiting from long range vocational programming. Unfortunately, many professionals working with the developmentally disabled have assumed that vocational training requires a high level of intelligence, an exorbitant amount of time for formal training, and an abundance of financial resources.

It is important to note that while many vocational programs do adhere to the above criteria, others serve clients who have a minimum of intelligence and operate programs which require a minimum amount of training time and financial resources. Gold (1969) has been successful in developing programs to teach complex vocational skills to trainable or moderately handicapped students. Many vocationally oriented jobs are available in the community, and require a minimum amount of training time. These jobs emphasize skills such as collating, color coding, sorting, assembling, filling envelopes, etc. Society has discouraged the developmentally disabled from volunteering for complex training programs and has offered them mundane, repetitive jobs which traditionally have not been of interest to the working population. Freidson (1965) describes a career for the handicapped as one which consists in large part of attempts to avoid a role rather than to play a role. The characteristic career of the handicapped often consists of a progressive narrowing of alternatives until none but the deviant or most unimportant role remains. In essence, the role that no one else wants. In terms of careers, the developmentally disabled are limited from the very beginning. Most handicapped individuals, especially the severely handicapped, have remained at home or in a school or facility until the age of 18 or 21 and have received, if any, very limited part time employment and training. At best, the goal was placement in a sheltered workshop which often was available only to a few students. Curriculum to prepare the developmentally disabled adolescent for a sheltered work environment has been conspicuously absent from most school programs. Bender and Valletutti (1976) have developed a total curriculum package that provides workshop oriented tasks in behavioral objective form. Selected examples of their objectives are included in Table 1.

In addition to vocationally oriented tasks and an exposure to functional academics, the needs of the developmentally disabled adolescent should include experiences in safety skills and consumer skills. Safety skills should concentrate on safety precautions in the home and community, while working, using transportation, purchas-

Table 1.    Selected workshop-oriented behavioral objectives

---

1. The student assembles parts of an object to make the whole object.
2. The student assembles parts of an object to make a section of the object.
3. The student disassembles small units of two or more parts.
4. The student separates continuous rolls of plastic sheeting, cloth, and bagging material into measured parts.
5. The student sorts by type, size, shape, and color of object.
6. The student inserts literature into envelopes for mailing.
7. The student inserts and packs assorted objects into a package.
8. The student sorts small objects using tweezers.
9. The student follows the directions provided with objects to be assembled.
10. The student uses simple diagrams to assemble objects.
11. The student socializes at breaks and other appropriate times.
12. The student works as a member of a group in the classroom, learning area, home, and job situation.

---

From Bender and Valletutti, 1976, vol. I, p. 260ff.

ing, cooking, eating and storing food, and while engaging in recreational activities. The teaching of consumer skills should emphasize the purchasing of goods and services and, when feasible, the use of banking facilities.

## PREVOCATIONAL EDUCATION

Prevocational education should be directly related to the field of work and is provided to give an individual the prerequisite skills and information required for entering the labor market. Prevocational education should be a major component of the curriculum for the developmentally disabled, but often it is not.

Traditionally, prevocational concepts begin with the introduction of topics involving the world of work. This would include people the students see or come in contact with on a regular basis such as their teachers, counselors, the school nurse, janitors, and cafeteria workers. Unfortunately, prevocational skills for most children are taught in isolation and often are not integrated into classroom routines. As an example, we often discuss the area of punctuality with the student and go through the myriad of rules which an employer would require. But, the student who comes in late to his class without an excuse often receives only a verbal reprimand without any other consequences.

It is also imperative that the teacher or professional working with the developmentally disabled adolescent serve as a good model at all times. When prevocational activities are available in the school curriculum it allows students to work together within a classroom setting. The ability to promote peer interaction and socialization is extremely important. Time is usually allowed for communicating with others within the classroom and offers an excellent opportunity for the teacher to observe the student exerting his independence. The importance of instituting prevocational activities before adolescence is critical. Many classroom jobs or situations can be arranged to give the students the necessary experience of working together or completing a project. Such activities would include being responsible for putting objects into their proper storage places after using them, potting plants, straightening books on the bookshelf, checking absentee lists, or, when feasible, telling the teacher what time it is at specific intervals during the day.

A major goal of the prevocational program is to serve as a prerequisite to a vocational program, and ultimately to provide the student with skills which will enable him to function as independently as possible in the community. Etienne and Morlock (1970) have described a prevocational program in Illinois where the objective was to have the mentally retarded client function independently in his community. In order to participate in the program, the students in this specific study received intensive training in the development of work skills and positive attitudes towards occupations, through a combination of classroom activities and job related experiences. It is important to note that the activities in the classroom were directly related to typical job experiences, and discussions represented what the student would be responsible for when he was on the job.

Often, the skills that the developmentally disabled have accumulated are not utilized in their eventual job placement. Many employers have stated they did not know the individuals possessed such skills. Educational and vocational assessment is therefore extremely critical and is presented in the following section.

## EDUCATIONAL AND VOCATIONAL ASSESSMENT

Educational and vocational assessment of the adolescent is critical if his special strengths and weaknesses are to be documented and an appropriate educational program is to be planned. Traditional educational assessments for the developmentally disabled have concerned themselves primarily with academic testing and not vocational evaluations. Often the student receives a specific grade equivalent score such as 2.3 which is interpreted as having skills equivalent to a student who is in the 3rd month of the 2nd grade. Little if any information is stated about the competencies or prevocational and vocational skills of the individual. A description of commonly used educational assessment instruments, and the academic areas they test is listed in Table 2.

A critical assessment of the developmentally disabled adolescent is the vocational evaluation which attempts to measure the individual's employment potential. Ideally, it should include tests to assess ability or aptitudes as well as those which indicate weak areas or limitations. One of the global goals of vocational evaluation has been to predict what the student might realistically expect to do in the world or work. There are many types of vocational processes. Some are conducted in a simulated employment environment which enables the evaluator to observe the reactions of students and their responses to demands that may be placed upon them in an employment situation.

Table 2.   Educational assessment instruments

| Name of test | Areas tested |
| --- | --- |
| California Achievement Test (CAT) | Vocabulary, reading comprehension, language, spelling, arithmetic |
| Detroit Test of Learning Aptitude | Pictorial-verbal absurdities, verbal-pictorial opposites, motor speed precision, auditory-attention span, visual attention span |
| Iowa Test of Basic Skills (ITBS) | Vocabulary, reading comprehension, language skills, work-study skills, arithmetic skills |
| Metropolitan Achievement Test | Word knowledge, word discrimination, reading, arithmetic, language |
| Peabody Individual Achievement Test (PIAT) | Arithmetic, reading recognition, reading comprehension, spelling, general information |
| Standard Achievement Test(s) | Word reading, paragraph meaning, vocabulary, spelling, word study skills, arithmetic, language |
| Wide Range Achievement test (WRAT) | Spelling, arithmetic, word pronunciation |
| Gates-McKillop Reading Diagnostic Test | Paragraph, phrase, word reading, letter sounds, auditory blending, syllabication, auditory discrimination, spelling |
| Gray Oral Reading Test | Oral reading |
| Key Math Diagnostic Arithmetic Test | Arithmetic skills (content, operations, and applications) |

Many vocational evaluation procedures involve a thorough psychometric testing, a work sample testing, and a critical observation of the student's behavior. The psychometric area is defined as the use of standardized tests to measure eye-hand coordination, gross manipulative ability, finger dexterity, mechanical ability, and form perception as well as interest inventories. An extensive sample of these instruments is included in Table 3.

Many programs and techniques are available for teaching the pre-vocational and vocational tasks that would be required in sheltered work or workshop programs. Techniques such as those advocated by Gold (1968) have emphasized that important considerations would include:

1. giving only one new item to learn at a time
2. adding a new step only after the old one has been thoroughly learned
3. analyzing any task to be taught and reducing it to the smallest possible steps

Another major component of vocational evaluation concerns itself with work samples. These can be defined as the combination of work tasks presented in an environment that is controlled and that simulates an actual work situation. The work samples usually are from actual jobs being performed in the community or in the workshop, and are graduated in difficulty. This phase of the evaluation is extremely important because it provides a concrete and positive demonstration whether or not the student is able to perform a task appropriately. At all times the evaluator is observing how the student is attempting to analyze the task and what previous knowledge he is applying to its solution. Notes are taken concerning the type of equipment or tools the student needs to use in order to complete the task. The rating of this phase of the vocational evaluation is based on a comparative completed task model.

The third component of the vocational evaluation concerns itself with observing the behavior of the student as he performs the task. Critical areas which are observed include the student's attention span, social skills, and his ability to accept and implement simple and complex directions. The entire vocational process including testing, work samples, and the observations of behavior all need to be analyzed critically if an accurate measure of the student's skills is to be accomplished. Currently systems which employ various facets of vocational evaluation have been utilized to work with those disabled students who

Table 3.   Vocational assessment instrument

| Name of test | Author and publisher | Purpose | Time to administer | Age level |
|---|---|---|---|---|
| Picture Interest Inventory | K. P. Weingarten California Test Bureau | To establish interest preferences and to group them in areas or clusters | 30–40 minutes | 7th grade to adult |
| Gordon Occupational Checklist | L. V. Gordon Harcourt Brace Jovanovich Inc. | A nonprofessional occupation interest inventory, to be used for counseling individuals interested in skilled, semi-skilled, and unskilled occupations | 20–25 minutes | High school age |
| Minnesota Vocational Interest Inventory (MVII) | K. E. Clark | A nonprofessional interest inventory; may be scored for 21 occupational scales (carpenter, plumber) and 9 general interest scales (ex. mechanical, health services, outdoor, etc.) | 45 minutes | Males 15 yrs. and older |
| Brainard Occupational Preference Inventory | P. P. and R. F. Brainard The Psychological Corporation | Assesses likes and dislikes and clusters them into professional interest area (ex. commercial, mechanical professional, scientific, agricultural, etc.) | 30 minutes | 8th–12th grade |
| Strong Vocational Interest Blank (SVIB) | E. K. Strong, Jr. Consulting Psychologists Press | To measure personal and occupational preferences and interests; for use in occupational counseling mainly for those planning to enter careers that require college education | 45 minutes | 16 and above |

| | | | | |
|---|---|---|---|---|
| Kuder Occupational Insterest Survey (OIS) | G. Frederic Kuder Science Research Associates | Compares person's responses to those of individuals in specific occupational groups (men: 72 occupational scales; women: 57 occupational scales, 29 college-major scales) for use in counseling placement, and job selection | 30 minutes | 9th to 12th grade and adult |
| Kuder General Interest Survey (GIS) | G. Frederick Kuder Science Research Associates | For use in vocational counseling in junior and senior high school; measures interest in ten general areas (ex. outdoor, mechanical, scientific, social service, clerical, etc.) | 45–60 minutes | 7th to 12th grade |
| Work Values Inventory (WVI) | D. E. Super Houghton Mifflin | Assesses 15 values that contribute to vocational success and occupational satisfaction | | 7th to 12th grade |
| Purdue Pegboard | J. Tiffin Science Research Associates | Measures manual dexterity and fine finger dexterity (indication of ability for assembly line or sheltered workshop tasks) | 5–10 minutes | Adolescent to adult |

*Continued*

Table 3—*Continued*

| Name of test | Author and publisher | Purpose | Time to administer | Age level |
|---|---|---|---|---|
| Pennsylvania Bi-Manual Worksample | J. R. Roberts American Guidance Service | Measures skills involving a combination of finger dexterity and gross arm and hand movements; for use in counseling students and adults choosing to enter industrial or mechanical occupations | As much time as needed to complete the task | |
| Minnesota Spatial Relations Test | M. R. Trabue, et al. American Guidance Service | Measures manual dexterity, space perception and mechanical comprehension | As much time as needed to complete the tasks | Jr. high to adult |
| Stromberg Dexterity Test | E. L. Stromberg The Psychological Corporation | Measures manual dexterity, speed and accuracy of finger, hand, and arm movements | As much time as needed to complete the tasks (usually 5–10 minutes) | Adolescent to adult |
| Test Of Mechanical Comprehension (TMC) | G. K. Bennett, et al. The Psychological Corporation | Measures mechanical ability, mechanical knowledge, and spatial ability | 30 minutes | |

have been in accidents and require rehabilitation. The TOWER System (Testing, Orientation, and Work Evaluation, and Rehabilitation), is an example of an evaluation procedure which may be utilized for the developmentally disabled.

## WORK STUDY

In the public school setting, many developmentally disabled adolescents take part in work-study programs. These programs allow the student to spend part of his day or week acquiring work experience and skills on special jobs that are available in the community, and then to return to school to learn the academic and vocational skills necessary for that specific job. Unfortunately, many special education teachers are trained to teach primary academic skills, and their classrooms reflect purely academic instruction with little emphasis on vocational evaluation, training, interviewing techniques, or other important career education areas. At times there is a lack of communication between the teacher and the vocational counselor. Too often the adolescent who successfully completes a work-study program may be trained for a job that is of interest to the teacher but is not available in the job market. Hammerlynck and Espeseth (1969) supported this view and reported sporadic and inadequate continuity of services as students progress through work-study programs. These factors, in addition to limited time to develop and supervise work experiences, and a lack of vocational educational skills in the special education teacher, have resulted in fewer jobs being offered to the developmentally disabled client. In 1972, Martin stressed the view that the educational system is just beginning to look at employment as an important subgoal of many programs. The developmentally disabled adolescent needs to have training in such areas as participation in an interview, completing an application, and, in some instances, searching for employment, as early in his program as possible.

Studies involving mentally retarded adolescents who have completed work study programs have offered some interesting observations. Job failure appears to be prevalant, not because of the mentally retarded's inability to do the work, but because of the failure of this individual to adjust to the social demands of the world of work (Gold, 1973). Knight (1972) concluded that there is some evidence that developmentally disabled individuals may at times be unrealistic in the establishment of their own vocational goals. Retarded children are generally aware that people work but are often unaware of what work means in terms of occupations that exist in our modern society. Many developmentally disabled adolescents, along with their teachers, do not thoroughly understand what requirements are necessary to fulfill many of the jobs they may be applying for in the near future. The need for appropriate educational programming for the adolescent developmentally disabled student cannot be overemphasized. Parents of handicapped students would agree that they want their children to become as independent as possible and to perform at an optimal level (Stanfield, 1973).

Parents are becoming more vocal in expecting that their adolescents be given training in social living as well as community living competencies. While the goal of performing some type of sheltered work is looked upon as a necessity for this population of students, the educational and vocational skills required to achieve this goal are often not taught in many school programs. When reasons for failure on job interviews for sheltered employment are assessed, the developmentally disabled adolescent characteristically has difficulty in certain areas (Nitzberg, 1974). These included:

1. fright, unable to answer questions
2. lack of exposure to this specific situation
3. failure to bring necessary papers to interviews such as social security information and so forth
4. had difficulty following questions on applications
5. refused to try any type of testing
6. had difficulty staying in the seat, was nervous
7. type of work applied for did not really interest them
8. failure to keep the appointment

Teaching special skills in interviewing, completing applications, and applying for jobs is of paramount importance and needs to be included in all curricula for developmentally disabled adolescents who eventually will be seeking employment (Bender and Valletutti, 1976).

## CONCLUSION

It is extremely critical that the developmentally disabled adolescent be prepared for maximal independence in the community. This preparation must start as early as possible. Job placement and socialization skills are mandatory requirements of their curricula. It is imperative that the special class teacher, vocational counselor, and other professionals work with the parents to monitor the student's performance in terms of his potential for success in later life. Historically, vocational preparation has been neglected in the education of the handicapped. Preparation for the world of work must now be a major component of the curricula for the developmentally disabled adolescent.

## REFERENCES CITED

Barclay, A. G., and L. Goulet. 1965. Short term changes in intellectual and social maturity of young noninstitutionalized retardates. Am. J. Ment. Defic. 70:257–261.

Bender, M., Valletutti, P., and Bender, R. 1976. Teaching the Moderately and Severely Handicapped, Volumes I, II, and III. University Park Press, Baltimore.

Braham, M. 1975. Peer Group Deterrents to Intellectual Development During Adolescence. In: R. Muuss (ed.), Adolescent Behavior and Society: A Book of Readings, pp. 256–264. Random House, New York.

Buckler, B. 1971. Living with a Mentally Retarded Child. Hawthorn Books, New York.

Carp, E. A. 1960. The world conception of the mentally deficient human being. J. of Existent. Psychiatr. Vol. I.

Child, I. L. 1953. Children Training and Personality: A Cross Cultural Study. Yale University Press, New Haven.

Collins, H., and G. Burger. 1970. The self concepts of adolescent retarded students. J. Ed. Train. Ment. Retard. 5:23–30.

Dittmann, L. 1959. The Mentally Retarded Child at Home. U.S. Dept. Health, Education and Welfare Social and Rehabilitation Service, Children Bureau Pub. #374. Washington, D.C.

Etienne, J. and Morlock, D. 1970. A pre-vocational program for institutionalized mental retardates. Train. School Bull. 67:228–234.

Farber, B. 1968. Mental Retardation: Its Social Context and Social Consequences. Houghton Mifflin, Boston.

Foale, M. 1956. The special difficulties of the high grade mental defective adolescent. Am. J. Ment. Defic. 60:867–877.

Freidson, E. 1965. Disability as social deviance. In: M. B. Sussman (ed.), Sociology and Rehabilitation, pp. 71–99. American Sociological Assoc., Washington, D.C.

Gold, M. 1968. Pre-workshop skills for the trainable: a sequential technique. J. Ed. Train. Ment. Retard. 3:31–37.

Gold, M. 1973. Research on the vocational habilitation of the retarded: The present, the future. In: N. R. Ellis (ed.), International Review of Research in Mental Retardation. Vol. 6. Academic Press, New York.

Hammerlynck, L. A., and Espeseth, V. K. 1969. Dual Specialist: Vocational rehabilitation counselor and teacher of the mentally retarded. Ment. Retard. 7:49–50.

Knight, O. B. 1972. Occupational aspirations of the educable mentally retarded. Train. School Bull. 69:54–57.

Lambert, B., Rothschild, B., Atland, R., and Green, L. 1972. Adolescence. Brooks/Cole, Monterey, Cal.

Martin, E. W. 1972. Individualism and behaviors as future trends in educating handicapped children. Except. Child. 38:517–525.

Mayer, C. L. 1966. The relationship of early special class placement and the self concepts of mentally handicapped children. Except. Child. 33:77–81.

McDaniel, C. O. 1970. Participation in extracurricular activities, social acceptance, and social rejection among educable mentally retarded students. J. Ed. Train. Ment. Retard. 5:4–14.

Muuss, R. 1975. Theories of Adolescence. Random House, New York.

Nitzberg, J. 1974. Why some students can't keep a job. J. Spec. Ed. Ment. Retard. 10:208–210.

Saenger, G. 1957. The adjustment of severely retarded adults in the community. In: H. Robinson and N. Robinson, The Mentally Retarded Child, p. 546. McGraw-Hill, New York.

Stanfield, J. S. 1973. Graduation: what happens to the retarded child when he grows up? Except. Child. 39:548–552.

# chapter eight
# DENTAL NEEDS
Beverly A. Entwistle, R.D.H., M.P.H.

The years of adolescence have been described by one author (Barber, 1969) as representing a dental revolution. Revolution, however, implies a sudden, radical, or complete change. This author prefers to characterize adolescence as a dental evolution, or a process of change—of unfolding and growing. During this period the adolescent begins to wean himself from his parents in terms of supervision of oral hygiene, dietary habits, responsibility for dental appointments, and a host of other activities, in an attempt to gain the independence of adulthood. The ways in which a developmental disability can alter the growth process have been outlined in other chapters. This chapter attempts to provide a framework from which professional nurses may determine the most appropriate manner of contributing to the dental health of developmentally disabled adolescents and young adults. The focus of this chapter is not on basic dental health information, but rather the provision of a framework for utilizing that knowledge when dealing with developmentally disabled individuals. The reader is referred to other references for a review of basic dental information (Fox, 1973, Colby, Kerr, and Robinson, 1971).

Developmentally disabled adolescents traditionally have been given little attention by the dental profession. Very little literature exists, therefore, that will prove to be beneficial to dental professionals or nondental professionals desiring increased knowledge of dental concerns. After working with numerous nondental professionals and developmentally disabled clients, this author is convinced that nondental personnel can provide a valuable contribution to the oral health of developmentally disabled adolescents.

## DENTAL NEEDS

At present there are no comprehensive epidemiological data on the dental conditions found in this particular population group. Most studies have included wide age ranges, thus providing a general overview of the conditions encountered in developmentally disabled individuals, but few are specific to adolescence. In an article by Hammer and Barnard (1966), 44 mentally retarded adolescents, the majority between ages 13 and 16, were studied to determine various characteristics of this age group. Specific dental conditions were not described, although it was noted that dental care was neglected. Whether the deteriorated dental status was due to an increased incidence of dental disease or lack of treatment for the disease cannot be determined from the reported study. Although no data are presented, Barber (1969) states that the dental conditions of handicapped individuals are no different from those observed in the normal population, yet may be aggravated by factors that will be discussed in later sections of this chapter. Snyder, Knapp, and Jordan (1960) support this view.

The obvious lack of data in the literature demonstrates the need for further epidemiological research regarding the dental conditions of developmentally disabled adolescents. In view of this lack of accurate data, specific dental conditions will be discussed in terms of the factors that may cause problems for developmentally disabled adolescents.

### Dental Caries

According to a national survey on health statistics (U.S. Dept. of Health, Education, and Welfare, 1974), the caries attack rate (decay rate) is higher during adolescence in normal populations than in any other age category. One factor contributing to this high rate is the eruption of a majority of the permanent posterior teeth during this time, which provides numerous newly erupted surfaces for bacterial attack (Massler, 1969). Concurrently, the teeth are subjected to a large amount of carbohydrates that provide a substrate for bacterial action. If the decay process is not arrested, gross dental caries can result, causing a severe dental and social problem for the growing adolescent.

The major contributing factors to severe dental caries attack in developmentally disabled adolescents appear to be the same as those affecting the normal population: 1) inadequate oral hygiene, 2) improper diet (high in fermentable carbohydrates), and 3) untreated carious lesions. The key to dealing with these factors is prevention, which includes early emphasis on good oral hygiene and eating habits, adequate fluoride intake, early detection of carious lesions, and prompt treatment. The benefits of optimal fluoride intake have been clearly documented (Horowitz, 1974). Determination of fluoride intake through topical or systemic ingestion for each individual is important. For families utilizing well water rather than water from municipal systems, public health departments will usually provide containers for water samples for analysis and determination of natural fluoride levels. Appropriate recommendations for receiving optimal benefits from fluoride can then be formulated.

Attitudes and behavior developed prior to adolescence will greatly determine the type of oral conditions with which the adolescent must contend. Developmentally disabled individuals do not need the additional burden of a dental disability that could have been prevented.

## Periodontal Disease

Inflammation of the gingival (gum) tissues has not usually been perceived as a childhood or adolescent dental problem by most people. Hormonal changes, poor nutrition, infection from untreated dental caries, malocclusion, and poor oral hygiene habits during adolescence, however, create a definite gingival problem for developmentally disabled individuals. The majority of these conditioning factors are amenable to treatment or oral hygiene therapy if these services are sought and maintained. An additional factor affecting the gingiva is the enlargement of gingival tissue caused by prolonged doses of the anticonvulsant drug phenytoin sodium (Dilantin) (Gurian, Ryan, and Daniels, 1975). In some instances scrupulous oral hygiene will partially alleviate the problem; in other cases gingival surgery is necessary. In certain cases gingival disorders are secondary to systemic diseases (e.g., leukemia) or prolonged antibiotic therapy that changes the oral flora (Wentz and Pollock, 1969).

## Occlusion

In childhood much of the developing occlusion may be based on genetic determination (Thompson, 1969). Environmental factors such as premature loss of teeth, abnormal muscular pressure, and disturbances in growth centers can, however, influence development and cause various orthodontic problems. Two primary factors that can determine whether an adolescent's mouth will be healthy or abnormal are the forces of deglutition and mastication. For developmentally disabled individuals who have inadequate muscle control or exaggerated tongue and lip habits, occlusion may be abnormal. Frequent bruxing or grinding of the teeth often occurs in deaf-blind individuals or those with cerebral palsy, and can create disturbances in occlusion or the temporomandibular joint. Orthodontic consultation should be considered for any individual manifesting such conditions. Early detection, interception, and guidance may occasionally be the only effective treatment where there are contraindications for full banded orthodontics (Owen and Graber, 1974). Although orthodontic treatment for improved dental health is the primary goal, treatment for cosmetic value should not be overlooked in individuals with a developmental disability, since appearance is as important to them as to any other individual.

Speech problems might accompany various types of malocclusion. In the majority of cases, however, correcting the dental problems will not automatically correct the speech problems, and parents and speech therapists should be made aware of this fact.

**Trauma**

Due to lack of muscular coordination or visual problems in some developmentally disabled individuals, fracturing of teeth and lip lacerations are not uncommon. These accidents should be referred to a dentist immediately, particularly if the tooth displays any discoloration. With the increasing interest in recreational activities for developmentally disabled individuals, additional safety precautions such as mouth guards for contact sports are advised. Injuries to the lip or oral tissues can also be observed in self-abusive individuals. A behavior modification approach, in addition to dental treatment, may be required to correct these habits. Orofacial trauma, manifested as burns, lacerations, bruises, and fractures, is also observed in up to one half of all reported cases of child abuse (ten Bensel and King, 1975). Post-operative injury to the lips, tongue, or oral mucosa caused by biting an anesthetized area is a definite concern of dental professionals. Caution should be taken to avoid this situation by frequent reminders to the adolescent and, if appropriate, to the guardian or residential worker, not to chew until normal sensation returns.

**Congenital Anomalies**

Occasionally, congenital anomalies such as cleft palate are the reason for a person's being labeled as developmentally disabled. In other cases, however, congenital craniofacial anomalies can occur secondarily to the major cause of the disability. Dental anomalies are frequently encountered in medical syndromes as in Down's syndrome,

Pierre-Robin syndrome, or congenital rubella (Gellis and Feingold, 1968). Some of the defects are skeletal, while others appear as defects in the tissues comprising the teeth. Various authors (Kraus, Clark, and Oka, 1968, Cohen and Diner, 1970) report increased incidence of enamel defects in mentally retarded and neurologically impaired individuals, indicating a relationship in the etiology of these developmental disturbances. Based on knowledge of patterns of dental development, these defects can sometimes be used as a gross diagnostic aid to determine the time at which the disturbance occurred.

## Medical Conditions

In addition to these specific dental conditions, numerous medical conditions or diseases exert pronounced effects on oral conditions or influence certain aspects of dental treatment. A comprehensive medical history, therefore, is normally required by dental professionals before rendering treatment to developmentally disabled individuals. Conditions frequently included in a medical history form are listed in Table 1.

Nursing professionals, with their extensive medical background, can assist in this endeavor by providing accurate and complete

Table 1.    Medical history: areas of concern to dental professionals

1. History of:
   a.  Heart murmur, congenital heart defect, rheumatic fever
   b.  Hypertension
   c.  Diabetes
   d.  Kidney disease
   e.  Respiratory disease or problems
   f.  Asthma
   g.  Seizures, convulsions
   h.  Blood disorders
   i.  Skin disease
   j.  Liver disease or problem
   k.  Other conditions
2. Allergies
3. Unusual reactions to medications
4. Present medications (type, frequency, dose)
5. Special diet
6. Fluoride intake
7. Name, address, phone number of physician; consent to obtain pertinent records
8. Date of last physical exam
9. Date of last dental exam

medical information and answering questions that may arise during the course of treatment. In view of the multiple medical problems of many developmentally disabled persons, dental professionals should be reminded to update their records frequently in terms of changes in medications or diet, hospitalizations, allergies, and numerous other factors.

Because nurses are often the primary health personnel who come in contact with developmentally disabled individuals as infants, and sometimes the only health professionals who deal with the individual as an adolescent, they can provide valuable assistance in case finding, referral, and follow-up. Unfortunately, the majority of nurses do not receive adequate education regarding dental health during their formal educational program. This lack of dental knowledge has become apparent in situations such as Early Periodic Screening, Diagnosis, and Treatment (EPSDT) programs, or school systems where nurses are responsible for dental screening. Although recognition overlaps diagnosis to a certain extent, nursing professionals should be prepared to recognize abnormal versus normal conditions in order to initiate referrals to dental professionals for a thorough diagnosis. Detection of suspected carious lesions is particularly important. All too frequently one encounters a report of gross caries, which in reality are chocolate cookie crumbs lodged in or around the teeth.

Oral inspections are frequently misused by school systems or residential institutions in that they are performed yearly on a mass basis to detect gross dental problems, without adequate follow-up regarding referral or treatment of the conditions. All dental screening should be performed for a specific purpose such as: 1) recording oral hygiene status in order to initiate a meaningful oral hygiene program, 2) recording baseline data to determine overall dental needs, 3) determining the extent to which previous problems received treatment, and 4) detecting dental problems in children not receiving regular dental care.

Most developmentally disabled adolescents cooperate for oral inspections provided that the procedure is carefully explained in terms of "just looking." Occasionally queries such as, "You're not going to pull my teeth, are you?" may arise. This fear should be immediately eliminated and time spent discovering why attitudes or past experiences prompted the fear, so that attempts at attitude change or dental treatment can be appropriately planned. Use of tongue blades to gain access to the mouth may sometimes trigger a psychological gag response in certain individuals. Self-retraction of lips and cheeks by the individual may be more effective than attempting to override the gag reflex.

To the adolescent the mouth is a sensitive area psychologically and emotionally as well as physically. Because of the numerous physical changes occurring during adolescence, body image is accentuated at this age (Daniel, 1970). Individuals may be shy or over-anxious about opening their mouths, especially if they feel that their dental condition is less than adequate. The emphasis that is placed on the "pearly white smile" by mass media and producers of commercial dental products can contribute to a lowered self-image if in fact his teeth do not conform to this image. If possible, the "pearly white" image should be de-emphasized and replaced by a more accurate image emphasizing cleanliness and function of teeth. The relationship of a "healthy" smile to overall health might be more appropriate.

## ORAL HYGIENE

The oral hygiene needs of developmentally disabled adolescents are frequently overlooked, yet they constitute a major dental problem. Oral hygiene is particularly important in terms of its relation to the development of dental caries and periodontal disease, and thus assumes the primary focus of preventive dentistry. In considering the various aspects of oral hygiene, it is essential that the nurse be able to differentiate between hard calculus (tartar) deposits and soft food debris in terms of their etiology, differences in methods of removal, and implications for dental health. What may initially appear to be a need for a professional dental prophylaxis may actually be a need for more thorough toothbrushing.

Once the oral conditions have been identified, one must assess their cause. The presence of heavy food debris, for example, may be due to: 1) lack of tongue control, 2) diet consisting of soft, adherent food, 3) lack of motor coordination to perform toothbrushing, 4) inadequate toothbrushing stroke, 5) infrequent attempts at oral hygiene care, or 6) untreated dental disease causing food impaction. Appropriate and effective means of dealing with this situation can only be instituted if all the causes of the problem are determined. For instance, no amount of clamoring for more frequent toothbrushing will alleviate the problem if the individual does not possess the motor coordination to perform adequate toothbrushing. Approaching these situations through the process of task analysis is extremely helpful. One such approach is outlined in Table 2, which presents the situation

Table 2.   Task analysis of a toothbrushing problem

1.   Does he have a toothbrush?
2.   Are the bristles soft and flexible or stiff?
3.   Can he identify the toothbrush?
4.   Does he know what and where his teeth are?
5.   Can he recognize the presence of food debris on his teeth?
6.   Can he adequately grasp the toothbrush?
7.   Does he have sufficient motor ability to produce a brushing motion?
8.   Does he have a bite or gag reflex?
9.   Can he squeeze the toothpaste on the brush in an appropriate amount?
10.  Can be brush all areas of his mouth?
11.  Does he consistently miss the same areas?
12.  Does he maintain attention long enough to complete the task?
13.  Can he repeatedly brush in the same sequence?
14.  Can he indicate how long he should be brushing?
15.  Can he differentiate between directional terms such as right, left, up, front?
16.  Does he correlate brushing with removing food and germs?

of the adolescent who does not brush his teeth. This list of questions can also be categorized in the following manner:

1.   Does he have the necessary equipment, and is it appropriate?
2.   Is he physically able to perform the task?
3.   Can he mentally comprehend the task and the directions?
4.   Does he possess the necessary attending and sequencing skills to adequately complete the task?

Based on this approach, one can arrive at appropriate solutions for individual problems rather than merely reiterating the need for brushing. In the case of an individual confined to a wheelchair, location of a sink which was accessible and at an appropriate level overcame a major barrier to oral hygiene (Figure 1). For those individuals who exhibit grasping problems, adaptation of toothbrushes in the form of thicker, longer, or bent handles may be necessary (Figure 2). If an adolescent is not capable of self-brushing due to his disability (e.g. quadriplegia, severe cerebral palsy), he must rely on others to accomplish the task (Figure 3). The adolescent should, however, be encouraged to do as much as he is physically capable of prior to intervention by another person. For those persons who cannot mentally comprehend the reasons for brushing, the task will have to be established as a habit. If verbal directions are not effective, physical demonstration and assistance may be needed. Frequently, when

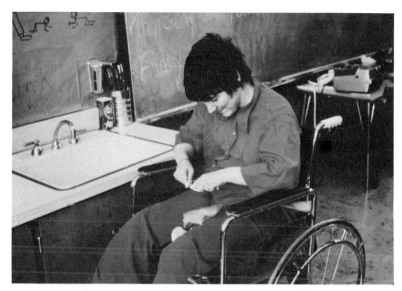

Figure 1.   Provision of appropriate equipment, such as a sink accessible from a wheel-chair, is a necessary step in promoting effective oral hygiene habits.

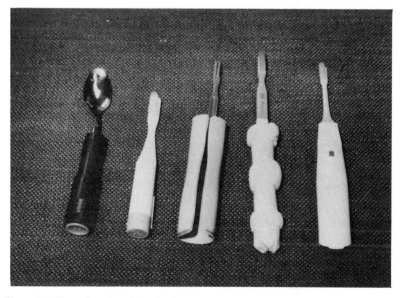

Figure 2.   Examples of toothbrush adaptations to accommodate individuals with grasping problems.

attending and sequencing skills are inadequate, supervision is required to make sure the task is completed.

The developmentally disabled adolescent may tend to be more conscious of personal appearance in an attempt to look more "normal." Due to the type of disability or lowered parental expectations, however, neatness may be a problem. Personal hygiene, which includes oral hygiene, should receive much emphasis at this age, since habits developed early will carry over into adulthood (Figure 4). Lack of muscular coordination or other factors can sometimes cause constant drooling. The social inappropriateness and methods of dealing with this situation (such as using a handkerchief) should be explained to the adolescent, so that he will not be needlessly embarrassed in social situations or excluded from certain types of employment such as food preparation.

Since nursing professionals frequently have a responsibility for providing health education, incorporation of dental health concepts in health education activities is greatly appreciated by dental professionals. One author (Tjossem, 1966) believes that motivated dental professionals provide more effective dental health education

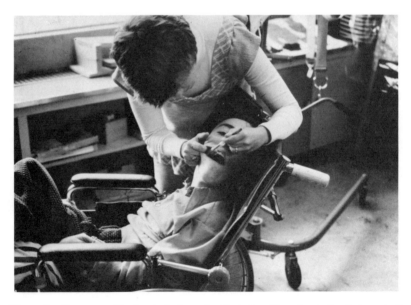

Figure 3. Proper positioning techniques facilitate brushing the teeth of those individuals incapable of self-brushing.

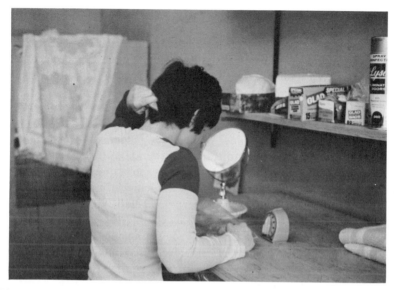

Figure 4.  Methods of oral hygiene care should be incorporated with other grooming skills in a home or school setting.

than school teachers or other nondental personnel. This author, however, believes that dental professionals may provide initial motivation and information to adolescent patients, but that informed and motivated teachers or residential workers who can provide daily reinforcement will be more effective in the long run.

When attempting to provide dental health education to developmentally disabled adolescents, nursing professionals may be frustrated by the lack of materials available for this age group. Although various professional dental organizations produce materials geared for all age groups and some minority groups, there are few materials appropriate for use with mentally retarded individuals. Mentally retarded adolescents pose a particular problem in that the language of the adult materials is too complex, while the more comprehensible materials are geared to younger age groups and thus portray inappropriate role models. There is a definite need, therefore, for development of dental health materials, particularly for physically handicapped and mentally retarded adolescents and adults. In view of the current lack of appropriate materials, nursing professionals may desire to create their own materials or adapt those already available.

## NUTRITION

Given the relation between diet and dental caries, nutrition is generally an integral part of dental health education. It is of particular concern during adolescence, since many of the "favorite snacks" consists of fermentable carbohydrates and empty calories. The food cravings that occur during adolescence can constitute a problem for those developmentally disabled individuals who are less active or who do not possess sufficient inner controls or judgment to curtail their eating habits. Often, both dietary and dental problems may be a reflection of the parents' inability to set appropriate and consistent expectations. Many school programs are currently initiating weight control programs for overweight developmentally disabled teenagers to teach them the fundamentals of acceptable eating habits. Dental personnel should be informed if any of their adolescent patients are on special diets so that the nutrition recommendations can be coordinated.

Although the food selection of developmentally disabled adolescents may be no different from that of other adolescents, they may be given a higher proportion of food rewards by parents, teachers, or therapists (Hammer and Barnard, 1966). Food rewards such as candy or cookies constitute a major dental problem when employed on a long term basis, as in some behavior modification programs. Crackers, pretzels, fruit, or nuts might be suggested as substitutes, provided that the individual's swallowing mechanisms are not seriously impaired. Gradually the food rewards should be discontinued and replaced by something more appropriate for a social or work setting, so that the adolescent will not expect to receive food rewards throughout his adult life.

## REFERRAL TO DENTAL PROFESSIONALS

Acquisition of dental treatment has proved to be a major roadblock in maintaining the dental health of developmentally disabled individuals. A frequent parental complaint has been, "I can't find a dentist who will treat my child. As soon as they hear a label such as mental retardation or cerebral palsy, they refer him to a specialist or to a hospital." Developmentally disabled adolescents are particularly neglected in this respect. Also, most adolescent clinics in hospitals do not provide dental services (Tjossem, 1966).

The term "adolescence" indicates "growing up," and these individuals literally grow out of the realm of pedodontics (children's dentistry) and into the realm of the general dentist. Pedodontists, in addition to treating children, have traditionally treated developmentally disabled patients, sometimes into adulthood. The majority of dental schools do not train the undergraduate dental students to treat this population group. Due to their busy schedules, however, pedodontists are becoming more reluctant to treat developmentally disabled adults, yet there are few other referral possibilities. The developmentally disabled adolescent, therefore, is stuck in the gap. This situation is especially distressing since the majority of developmentally disabled individuals can be treated successfully in private practice or clinic settings rather than under general anesthesia in a hospital.

An attempt has been made to alleviate this problem by the creation of 10 programs in 1974 funded by the Robert Wood Johnson Foundation to train undergraduate dental and dental hygiene students to deal with individuals of all ages who are developmentally disabled (Nowak, 1974). These programs are still too young to determine their effectiveness. Hopefully, as a result of these programs, access to care will be more available to developmentally disabled adolescents.

In addition to these undergraduate training programs, various government sponsored University Affiliated Programs for the developmentally disabled provide training for undergraduate and graduate students as well as community professionals regarding the dental needs of this population. There are 47 such centers across the nation which operate on an interdisciplinary model of diagnostic, treatment, and consultation services for developmentally disabled persons and the agencies that serve them. These centers have often proved helpful to nurses desiring further information on training in the area of developmental disabilities.

Nurses will discover that the most successful referral process entails knowing the local resources and who will accept what types of patients under what conditions. A referral list can then be developed from this information with frequent updating at specified intervals.

## FINANCIAL CONSIDERATIONS

Federal priorities for dental health programs in the United States have primarily emphasized dental care for children. Presently, Federal support declines when an individual reaches age 21, even if a developmental disability is present. Medicaid's "over 21" dental coverage, when available, usually only includes emergency services or denture fabrication with few provisions for preventive or restorative services. The paucity of dental insurance for adults, therefore, makes it even more important that developmentally disabled adolescents receive most of their primary care before adulthood, so that only maintenance and preventive services are necessary after that time. If, as an adult, the individual is declared his own legal guardian and receives his income from an income maintenance program such as Supplemental Security Income or Social Security, financing dental care is extremely difficult, based on the meager spending money that remains after basic living expenses. Given their limited financial resources, it is understandable that dentistry is given low priority consideration.

## TRANSPORTATION AND OFFICE ACCESSIBILITY

If a developmentally disabled adolescent is living in a group home or other community living facility, transportation can be difficult, especially if home operators do not provide transportation for the residents. Public transportation, if available, is an additional financial burden and may not transport the person directly to the location of his appointment. Some developmentally disabled individuals do not possess the skills to utilize public transportation.

Physically handicapped persons who are in wheelchairs encounter additional transportation problems when scheduling dental appointments. Most types of public transportation do not accommodate wheelchairs. Many dental offices or clinics are located in buildings inaccessible to wheelchairs because of staircases or crowded conditions. Dental operatories may also not be adaptable to wheelchairs or permit transfer of heavy individuals to the dental chair. When calling for an appointment, these factors should be considered by both the dental personnel and the handicapped individual.

## DENTAL APPOINTMENTS

With the present national emphasis on deinstitutionalization, adolescents and young adults are being released from institutions to be reintegrated into community living. Frequently, these people have not been taught the necessary skills to function in a semi-independent fashion in the community. Often they do not possess the skills to locate a dentist who will accept them as a patient, to schedule an appointment, or to provide the necessary preliminary information that is required before dental services can be delivered. They will need assistance in these endeavors, along with training in handling similar situations in the future. All too often the assistance is provided but not the training. The developmentally disabled adolescent who lives at home could very well be in a comparable situation; the parents might be overprotective to the point of "doing rather than teaching," or the individual might have been infantalized so that he is unwilling to relinquish his dependency state. The end result is the same—developmentally disabled adolescents who are unprepared for independence and assumption of adult roles. In some cases this dependency state is reinforced by dental professionals who underestimate or overestimate the abilities of developmentally disabled individuals. The majority of these inappropriate expectations are probably the result of a lack of knowledge regarding how to access these abilities. Nurses can facilitate development of meaningful relationships between dental professionals and developmentally disabled adolescent patients in a variety of ways. In an attempt to provide a framework for doing this, various attitudes, behaviors, and actions that may occur during dental appointments will be discussed.

Upon entering the dental office, the adolescent can recognize cues that place him in a childlike or dependent position: reliance upon the accompanying adult for completion of medical history forms, discussion of procedures, and scheduling future appointments; voice intonations geared for a younger child. Inclusion of the adolescent in making decisions regarding his dental needs is one area that is particularly overlooked. Those individuals who manifest physical disabilities but are of normal intelligence encounter countless difficulties in this area due to a common misconception that a physical disability implies mental dysfunctioning.

Other actions or behaviors may accentuate the developmentally disabled person's feelings of being "different." Certain dental offices only schedule appointments for their "special patients" at specified times during the day or place the patients in individual dental operatories or "quite rooms." Although the stated purpose of these actions is to devote more time and attention to the individual, they are frequently done to avoid interaction between the regular patients and the "special patients." These actions and attitudes are certainly not conducive to the process of normalization, either from the standpoint of the disabled individual's integration into society or society's acceptance of the disabled individual. In certain instances, however, such as extreme embarrassment on the part of the patient, separation with gradual integration into the normal office routine may be advised.

Various problems that may occur revolve around socially sensitive issues about which people are generally uncomfortable. Inappropriate social behavior between professionals and disabled adolescents in the form of hugging, holding hands, and flirting is usually handled by the professional in one of two ways: 1) repulsion and rejection, or 2) return of affection as if it were delivered by a younger child. The former reaction is one that can only be dealt with by the professional himself. The latter is a reaction that should be discouraged, since it reinforces the behavior and provides inappropriate role models for socialization into adulthood. Occasionally, dental professionals are embarrassed by developmentally disabled patients who seemingly are masturbating while in the dental chair. Often this action is merely a signal that the person is in need of a rest room. If, in fact, the patient is masturbating, the nursing professional who is versed in concepts of human sexuality may be the most appropriate person to provide guidance on the issue for both the professional and disabled patient.

The relationship between the dental professional and the patient is the major determinant of a successful dental appointment. In the case of the developmentally disabled adolescent, feelings and emotions on both sides, whether expressed or unexpressed, are an integral part of this relationship. The dental professional may experience varied reactions to the disabled adolescent: repulsion, fear, sympathy, frustration. The adolescent, in turn, may feel self-conscious, fearful, frustrated, angry, or insulted. Unless both of these individuals deal with their feelings in some manner (e.g., discussion, desensitization), a meaningful dental relationship can never develop. All too often the dentist reacts by refusing to treat people with certain disabilities, while the disabled individual reacts by refusing to seek further dental care. Communication and understanding, therefore, are essential to provision and acceptance of dental care.

Certain procedures inherent to dental appointments may create problems for developmentally disabled adolescents. The supine position of most dental chairs creates the feeling of helplessness with no avenues for escape. Feelings of being in control of situations may be important for these individuals, since loss of control is too threatening and subconsciously implies further deviance. Introduction of countless instruments, suction apparatus, and other dental materials intraorally can create sensations of suffocation, particularly if the person's swallowing is impaired. Intraoral treatment also eliminates one avenue of communication, which is threatening for individuals who are blind or dependent upon verbal communication. In such instances an alternate communication or signal system might be developed by the dental staff and patient. Various noises that accompany dental treatment are especially frightening for those people with visual impairments or wearing hearing aids and should be introduced gradually with careful explanation. The auditory and visual distractions encountered during dental appointments can be a problem for hyperactive or easily distractible adolescents.

The provision of quality dental treatment requires extreme cooperation from the patient in terms of sitting still and maintaining attention; any excess movement can prove hazardous and time consuming. In the case of individuals manifesting cerebral palsy, this aspect is of major concern to dental professionals and may require modifications in treatment techniques, such as use of mouth props or physical restraints. Nursing professionals and dental professionals should recognize that dental appointments involve multiple stimuli that create difficulties for developmentally disabled individuals who cannot deal with more than a limited number of stimuli at one time. Careful preparation of these individuals before the appointment, as well as clear explanations and elimination of unnecessary stimuli during the appointment, will facilitate dental treatment for them.

In response to an overload of new stimuli that he is unable to organize, the developmentally disabled adolescent may lose control and engage in some types of acting out behavior. This behavior does not necessarily constitute a problem, provided the dentist understands the behavior and can control or modify it through use of verbal communication, psychosedation, or physical restraint. More importantly, the dentist may differentiate this type of behavior from that of a rebellious adolescent who is testing limits, since the origin of the behavior is different and requires different management techniques. It is interesting to note that professionals' and parents' perceptions of behavior problems are usually not the same (Hammer and Barnard, 1966). Parents' concerns are frequently expressed in terms of their child's negative behaviors—biting, not opening the mouth, not sitting still, screaming, not paying attention—usually behaviors that the parents themselves cannot control. They tend to be more concerned about the dentist's safety than the adolescent's. Dentists, on the other hand, usually perceive behavior problems in terms of their own inability to handle the situation. Emphasis should be placed on the development of appropriate behavior and positive attitudes rather than on punishment of inappropriate behavior. Inappropriate behavior, therefore, should often be ignored, and appropriate behavior highly reinforced. Problems occur, however, when the adolescent perceives different expectations and receives inconsistent or conflicting reinforcers from parents or dental professionals.

Nursing professionals can play an important role in developing and reinforcing appropriate dental behavior and attitudes, particularly during health education activities. Group sessions with peers are sometimes more effective, since adolescents are very amenable to group pressure (Tjossem, 1966). Because of traditional impressions or previous traumatic experiences, adults should assess their own attitudes and dental behavior and avoid transferring any negative attitudes to others. Frequently, developmentally disabled adolescents are programmed with negative attitudes prior to any actual dental visits so that acting out behavior is inevitable.

## FOLLOW-UP

No amount of dental treatment or health education is effective without a monitoring or follow-up system to reinforce proper attitudes and prevent occurrence of future problems. Unfortunately, follow-up care appears to be inadequate in most cases. All too often restorative care is provided until age 18, after which dental care is sought primarily on an emergency basis. In the case of group homes or residential facilities, records of dental visits or treatment performed are sorely lacking. Nursing professionals provide a vital communication link between developmentally disabled adolescents, institutional or residential workers, parents, educators, dental professionals, and other health professionals (Figure 5).

A professional who can coordinate and communicate dental health information and resources is greatly needed—someone who can place dental health in its proper perspective as a portion of total health care. This author believes that the nursing professional can effectively fulfill this function and actively advocate improved dental health for the developmentally disabled adolescent. For additional suggestions as to how nurses can provide this orientation, the reader is referred to an article by Smith (1970), which describes a successful dental program involving nursing personnel.

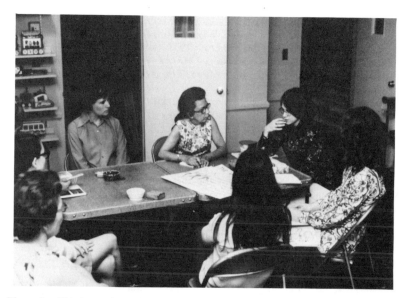

Figure 5.   This in-service training session scheduled by the school nurse, involved a discussion of basic dental health concepts and coordination of efforts among dental professionals, school staff and parents.

Although this chapter has attempted to outline various dental needs and aspects of dental care for developmentally disabled adolescents, a plethora of information is still unwritten. It is the hope of this author that this chapter will provide incentive and guidance for nursing professionals who have the opportunity to work with developmentally disabled adolescents.

## REFERENCES CITED

Barber, T. K. 1969. The handicapped adolescent. Dent. Clin. N. Am. 13:287–320.

Cohen, H. J., and Diner, H. 1970. The significance of developmental dental enamel defects in neurological diagnosis. Pediatrics 46:737–47.

Colby, R. A., Kerr, D. A., and Robinson, H. B. G. 1971. Color Atlas of Oral Pathology, 3rd. ed. J. P. Lippincott, Philadelphia.

Daniel, W. A. 1970. Adjustment to handicapping conditions. In: W. A. Daniel (ed.), The Adolescent Patient, pp. 339–344. C. V. Mosby, St. Louis.

Fox, L. A. 1973. Preventive dentistry for the handicapped child. Pediatr. Clin. N. Am. 20:245–258.

Gellis, S. S., and Feinfold, M. 1968. Atlas of Mental Retardation Syndromes. U.S. Government Printing Office, Washington, D.C.

Gurian, S., Ryan, P., and Daniels, E. 1975. Gingival hyperplasia due to dilantin therapy. J. Dent. Handicapped 1(3):11–17.

Hammer, S. L., and Barnard, K. E. 1966. The mentally retarded adolescent. Pediatrics 38:845–857.

Horowitz, H. S. 1974. Caries prevention and fluoride preparations. In: A Picozzi and J. Smudski (eds.), Pharmacology of Fluorides, pp. 36–43. First Symposium, I.A.D.R., Atlanta.

Kraus, B. S., Clark, G. R., and Oka, S. W. 1968. Mental retardation and abnormalities of the dentition. Am. J. Ment. Def. 72:905–917.

Massler, M. 1969. Teen-age cariology. Dent. Clin. N. Am. 13:405–423.

Nowak, A. J. 1974. Dental health for the mentally retarded citizen—Our shared concern. J. Dent. Handicapped 1(1):3–12.

Owen, D. G., and Graber, T. M. 1974. The developing occlusion–orthodontic considerations for the handicapped. Dent. Clin. N. Am. 18:711–721.

Smith, R. G. 1970. Meeting the challenge of dental care for retarded and physically handicapped children. Ment. Retard. 8:7–11.

Snyder, J. R., Knapp, J. J., and Jordon, W. A. 1960. Dental problems of non-institutionalized mentally retarded children. Northwest Dent. 39:23–33.

ten Bensel, R. W., and King, K. J. 1975. Neglect and abuse of children: Historical aspects, identification, and management. J. Dent. Child. 42:16–26.

Thompson, J. R. 1969. Dentofacial growth in the adolescent. Dent. Clin. N. Am. 13:343–354.

Tjossem, T. B. 1966. Psychological considerations in the case of the adolescent dental patient. Dent. Clin. N. Am. July: 449–461.

U.S. Dept. of Health, Education, and Welfare. 1974. Decayed, Missing and Filled Teeth Among Youths 12–17: United States. U.S. Government Printing Office, Washington, D.C.

Wentz, F. M., and Pollock, R. J. 1969. Periodontics. Dent. Clin. N. Am. 13:495–508.

# chapter nine

# NUTRITION AND NUTRITION EDUCATION NEEDS

Mary Helen Greenwood, M.S., R.D.

Meeting nutrition and nutrition education needs can be a challenge during adolescence. Unprecedented growth demands require high intakes of many nutrients and knowledge of how to obtain these nutrients. Further, many adolescents are exposed for the last time to classroom education that can aid them in becoming successful adults, living independently in the community. Knowing how to choose foods wisely, within budget and time constraints, must be an integral part of this education.

Most developmentally disabled adolescents are no different in their nutritional requirements from typical adolescents. Many mildly retarded adolescents also have the same aspiration of independent living as other adolescents. However, whether or not they will be able to live successfully and independently as adults depends in part upon receiving appropriate nutrition information. The importance of such education cannot be overemphasized for any developmentally disabled adolescent, as food and nutrition decisions will ultimately be reflected in his health, employability, and home and family adjustments.

It is hoped that nurses and others in various settings will encourage and plan appropriate nutrition education for developmentally disabled adolescents. The information provided in this chapter should serve as a basis for assessing nutritional needs and planning and carrying out nutrition education.

In this chapter, the term "developmentally disabled adolescents" refers to those individuals who may be handicapped by their physical maturity, physical disabilities, social maturity, and cognitive abilities. These disabilities may or may not affect their nutrition and nutrition education needs, but they certainly will affect the approach to discovering and meeting these needs.

The factors which affect adolescent nutrition requirements are too vast for complete coverage in one chapter. Further, it is equally important to consider the nutrition education needs of this population. Therefore, this chapter offers a general discussion of both nutrition and nutrition education for developmentally disabled adolescents, and then suggests a specific approach to assessing and planning for these needs. The purposes of this chapter are to:

1. acquaint the reader with important aspects of growth that have nutritional implications, the major adolescent nutritional needs, common problems seen in adolescence and how to avoid them, and how developmentally disabled adolescents may vary
2. offer a practical approach to the assessment of the nutritional status of developmentally disabled adolescents
3. increase the awareness of the nutrition education needs of these adolescents and to offer general guidelines for the assessment and planning of nutrition education needs
4. offer a specific outline showing how nutrition education should progress in the clinical, community, home, institutional, and group home settings

## DISTINGUISHING BETWEEN "NUTRITION" AND "NUTRITION EDUCATION"

There are many possible definitions of nutrition. Simply defined, nutrition concerns the nutrients in the food and water an individual eats and drinks and how his body uses them for maintenance, growth, activity, reproduction, and lactation. Nutrition is a science and should be based on properly executed and continuing scientific research.

Nutrition education is an educational process based on what is understood and believed about nutrition. It can be defined as "the process by which beliefs, attitudes, and understandings about food lead to habits that are nutritionally sound, practical, and consistent with individual needs and available food resources" (Todhunter,

1969). To provide optimal health through diet is the goal of nutrition education.

One important difference between nutrition and nutrition education is that nutrition is defined in terms of individual requirements, but does not assign responsibility for meeting those requirements. In some settings, the individual has little control over his own food intake. Nutrition education, on the other hand, implies involvement of the individual in an educational process that leads to improvement of his own diet habits.

## GROWTH AT ADOLESCENCE

Adolescents experience the second and final rapid physical and mental growth period of their lives. In girls this occurs at about 8 to 14 years of age and for boys at about 9 to 15 years of age (Mayer, 1972). The rapid growth demands greatly increased intake of most nutrients.

Unlike the child in the rapid growth phase during the neonatal period, adolescents may make many of their own food choices and may express their feelings, needs, and desires through these choices. The rapid growth and increased independence of adolescence makes this an essential time to offer nutritious food to meet growth requirements and nutrition education to encourage the individual to take responsibility for meeting his own growth needs.

### Clues to Growth Stage and Nutritional Needs

The onset, duration, and extent of the adolescent growth spurt varies from individual to individual. Whereas nutritional requirements in other phases of the life cycle may be closely related to age, this is not the case in adolescence. One cannot assume that all 14-year-olds, for example, need the same number of calories because one may be in the last stages of growth while another may be in the midst of the most rapid growth. In general, girls begin adolescence about 2 years earlier than boys.

The growth events do follow a definite sequence, closely related to the growth and development of the reproductive system. By following the growth and development of the reproductive system then, one can determine whether or not an adolescent has experienced the most rapid phase of linear growth, when energy and some nutrient requirements are greatest. Sexual maturity ratings (SMR) are an invaluable tool for estimating nutritional requirements (Tanner, 1962).

The nurse can ask a girl or care giver if the girl has begun menstruation yet. If not, then the girl is in the early stages of puberty and will be experiencing the adolescent growth spurt very soon. If menarche has already occurred, she has already experienced her growth spurt.

Boys do not have a definite indicator of development. In general one can look at an adolescent boy and note such things as muscular development, amount of hair on his upper lip, and the tone of his voice. If he does not appear "filled out," has little hair on his upper lip, and his voice has not deepened, he is probably in SMR 3. This indicates the rapid growth period and greatly increased nutrient needs.

### Assure Adequate Nutrition Throughout Adolescence

Growth does not cease after the rapid phase of growth; it only slows down. Huenemann et al (1974) noted the continuing growth in 9th through 12th grade boys and girls, even after their growth spurts. In boys, there was an increase in diameter, lean body weight, and stature, indicating skeletal growth, but also increasing circumference in their arms, calves, and biceps, indicating continued muscle growth. The girls increased in lean body weight, stature, and some diameters, though all increases were smaller than in boys.

### Timing of the Growth Spurt and Development of Obesity

There is a relationship between the timing of the growth spurt and the development of obesity. That is, those who mature early have a more intense growth spurt and after growth slows, may become obese. These individuals tend to be larger before adolescence and then heavier, but not taller after their growth slows. It is important to try to prevent excessive weight gain in early maturers, whenever possible.

### Summary

In summary, growth at adolescence is unique due to its rapidity, individuality, and finality. Nutrition is only one of the many factors affecting the timing, duration, and extent of growth, but it is probably the most important factor. In relation to nutritional needs, it is important to realize that growth does not cease after the adolescent spurt, but rather may continue even up to the thirtieth year of life and longer. Because growth varies widely from person to person, it is best to consider each person's developmental or biological age rather than chronological age in determining nutritional or other needs.

Developmentally disabled adolescents as other adolescents are interested in and concerned about growth. Those who are able to should have an understanding about growth and its characteristics.

## NUTRITIONAL REQUIREMENTS DURING ADOLESCENCE

While growth has been extensively studied and reported (Tanner, 1962), nutritional needs during adolescent growth are not well delineated. Two books (Heald, 1969, and McKigney and Munro, 1976) are collections of investigators' work in this area, but they by no means provide definitive information. Perhaps this is due to a lack of concentrated study in this area, but it is undoubtedly in part due to the wide range of individual variation in growth, its characteristics, and the nutrients needed to meet growth needs. Also, the possibility must be left open that there are nutritional requirements important for growth that have not yet been discovered. Further, there may be approaches to the assessment of nutritional needs that will update our knowledge, as pointed out in the last section of the book edited by McKigney and Munro (1976).

Historically, the determination of nutritional requirements has relied on the correction of a nutritional deficiency. But during growth, with the addition of more cells and an increase in the size of cells, one cannot rely on the correction of a deficiency as the sole determinant of nutrition requirements. Growth deficits due to nutritional deficiencies may not be obvious. The determination of "optimal" or "normal" intakes of nutrients for growth, maintenance, activity, and reproduction in adolescence is very difficult to define.

The nutritional health of adolescents depends on the nutrient supply to the cells as a function of their need. However, nutrition is part of a total health picture, and one must consider many factors that may affect the supply of nutrients to and their use by the cells. Environmental, physical, biological, and social factors also affect nutritional requirements.

The "Recommended Dietary Allowances" of the National Research Council (1973) are mentioned several times as a guide. These recommendations are revised about every 3 to 4 years and are useful as a guide to nutritional needs for various age groups. However, these recommendations must be used as a guide only. They are not a strict standard because they suffer from the same lack of information as any other source and are only general estimates. Also, needs are expressed according to age, which is not a good standard during the adolescent years. Still, these guidelines are useful to present the general picture of nutritional needs and as an easy reference. Table 1 presents a portion of the 1973 Recommended Dietary Allowances.

The best estimation of nutrient requirements depends on individual assessment. Where possible, each adolescent's growth, health status, present nutrient intake, and environmental factors should be assessed. Then, nutrient requirements can be estimated for the individual based on the general information discussed below.

During the peak of the adolescent growth spurt, requirements for calories, and minerals exceed needs both earlier and later. During this time, linear growth may be as much as .25 mm per day and the skeleton may gain 1.2 gram of dry weight per day (Garn, Wagner, 1969). Nutritional needs are also important before and after the rapid growth period. Adequate nutrition before the growth spurt helps assure that there will be no delay. Adequate nutrition is needed after the most rapid growth because though growth slows, it does not cease.

**Calories**

Because the growing body needs a lot of energy, it is important to look at "energy balance" or energy intake minus energy output in the growing adolescent. Obviously, energy is derived from foods in the form of potential energy: carbohydrates, fats, and protein. Space does not permit a complete discussion of energy balance. Of importance, however, is that for growth to occur over long periods of time, energy balance must be positive (Cooke, 1969). There is individual variation in stages of growth, activity level, body size, and body losses of energy. Some severely disabled adolescents whose physical activity is quite limited require energy needs that are less than normal.

Girls generally go through their peak growth 2 to 3 years earlier than boys. Therefore, their peak caloric needs normally occur earlier than those of boys. Further, in considering body size and need, the needs of boys are greater because they grow taller and gain more weight than girls.

One can refer to the Recommended Dietary Allowances (1973), but this is not enough in considering caloric needs. The best way to ascertain whether or not caloric needs are being met for growth, is to follow each individual's height and weight over time. By plotting height and weight on a standardized chart, one has the best indication of calorie status. One should also consider the caloric content of foods

Table 1. Food and Nutrition Board, National Academy of Sciences—National Research Council Recommended Daily Dietary Allowances[a]; Selected nutrients needed during adolescence (1973–1974)

| Sex | Ages | Energy (kcal) | Protein (g) | Vitamin A (I.U.) | Vitamin D (I.U.) | Ascorbic acid (mg) | Folacin (μg) | Calcium (mg) | Iron (mg) | Zinc (mg) |
|---|---|---|---|---|---|---|---|---|---|---|
| Males | 11–14 | 2,800 | 44 | 5,000 | 400 | 45 | 400 | 1,200 | 18 | 15 |
| | 15–18 | 3,000 | 54 | 5,000 | 400 | 45 | 400 | 1,200 | 18 | 15 |
| | 19–22 | 3,000 | 52 | 5,000 | 400 | 45 | 400 | 800 | 10 | 15 |
| Females | 11–14 | 2,400 | 44 | 4,000 | 400 | 45 | 400 | 1,200 | 18 | 15 |
| | 15–18 | 2,100 | 48 | 4,000 | 400 | 45 | 400 | 1,200 | 18 | 15 |
| | 19–22 | 2,100 | 46 | 4,000 | 400 | 45 | 400 | 800 | 18 | 15 |

[a] Food and Nutrition News, 1973–74. Vol. 45, no. 2, Dec.–Jan.

consumed by questioning the adolescent, his parent or caregiver, or observing intake at mealtime.

### Development of Obesity

In addition to early maturers, others are at risk for developing obesity. Those whose parents are obese, and adolescent females in general, are at risk because they add subcutaneous fat at a rapid rate during adolescence.

Some investigators have shown that overfeeding in rats during the growth period results in the adipose tissue responding by a sharp increase in the number of fat cells. In adult rats, the response is not an increase in number, but only in size. These extra fat cells are not lost when a normal intake is resumed in adolescence. Therefore, if this is also applicable to the human, overeating during the adolescent growth period may lead to irreversible obesity or obesity highly resistant to treatment.

It is best to attempt to prevent obesity by counseling individuals at risk to control their eating habits and by assuring that foods offered to these individuals are appropriate. Adolescents who can understand it should have the growth process explained to them. Further, for very young overweight adolescents, those who have not yet experienced their growth spurt, it should be pointed out that there is a possibility that by not overeating, they have a chance to grow into a more acceptable, thinner size. These individuals should be followed closely and should be encouraged to participate in their own diet and growth monitoring as much as possible.

Obesity can be determined by plotting height and weight on a standardized growth chart. Weight that is two standard deviations greater than height indicates obesity. Obesity also can be determined by taking arm circumference measures and skinfold thickness measures with a caliper and comparing the obtained values with standardized values.

During the growth spurt, calories should not be restricted so that weight is lost because this may hinder the individual from gaining his or her full growth potential. If however, it can be documented that the individual has passed the most rapid stage of growth, calorie restriction is warranted. By looking at dietary intake, it is usually fairly easy to determine problem foods and inappropriate intakes. The adolescent should be counseled, along with his parents or caregiver, about foods to eliminate or decrease. Emotional reasons for overeating should be explored, as well as the general emotional tension in the home that may be causing the adolescent to express his feelings through eating. Further, one must consider the adolescent's motivation to lose weight. It may be that, initially, the adolescent will not be interested in changing eating habits, but may be at a later visit. Weight loss success requires motivation from the adolescent and a willingness to control food intake.

One should also consider other environmental factors that may be adding to the weight problem. In institutions and group homes, it may be that foods served are high in calories. The adolescent may not be able to get plainly prepared foods and/or foods that are lower in calories such as skim milk and fruit. If this is the case, changes must be made in the food service.

## Protein Needs

Protein needs can be estimated in many ways. As with calories, there are no exact or even close estimates of protein needs in adolescence. Calorie intake must be adequate in order to keep protein from being used for energy rather than its primary function of tissue building. It is not known, however, whether or not extra protein is needed for the growth spurt in adolescence. Protein needs are considered to be greater for males than for females, because males have greater body size and muscle mass. There are greater needs for protein during infectious illness, injury, and surgery.

Nitrogen retention studies indicate that protein should constitute about 15% of the caloric intake (Johnston, 1958). This is only a guide, but probably an accurate one. Dietary intake studies have shown that adolescents consume protein in amounts from 12 to 14% of the caloric intake (Heald, Remmell, and Mayer, 1969). Further, adolescents appear to increase their protein intake during the growth spurt, although there is no present evidence to indicate that this is necessary (Hegsted, 1974).

Again, the best indicators of adequate protein intake are growth measures and food intake information. In examining food intake information, one should look for the quantity and quality of protein. Proteins vary in their quality or essentiality for growth and maintenance, but one should not forget to count those of poorer quality as contributing to the total protein intake. Those of high quality are meat, eggs, fish, milk, and milk products, and soybeans. Those of poorer quality come from grains and vegetables, but when they are combined in dishes with a small amount of high quality protein, a much greater overall value is obtained.

The protein intake of healthy adolescents is normally adequate or excessive, but may not be in abnormal or disease states.

### Fat Intake and the Development of Coronary Heart Disease

Adequate fat intake is normally of little concern in adolescence. Rather, there is currently much concern over excessive intakes of certain types of fat in adolescence, especially for certain "at risk" individuals. High consumption of saturated fats (those of animal origin) are a prime cause of elevated plasma cholesterol which is a major risk factor in coronary heart disease (Hegsted, 1976). There are some individuals who hereditarily are at risk for the development of coronary heart disease and these individuals particularly need to watch consumption of saturated fats.

Available data on intakes is sparse. However, it appears that while girls' intakes of fat peak and level off at about 12 to 14 years of age, boys' intakes increase until about age 18. Boys, then, appear to be a greater risk for excessive consumption of fat, though it is not known whether this would necessarily be saturated fat.

While individual assessment for coronary heart disease risk is best, it should also be pointed out that institutions and group homes may need to consider the fat content and type in meals served to residents. Currently, many new products are available to decrease consumption of saturated fat and increase consumption of unsaturated fat. In particular, the amount of beef, eggs, whole milk and milk products served should be considered. Further, margarines high in polyunsaturated fats could replace butter or margarines high in saturated fat.

For residents or individuals found to be at risk for the development of coronary heart disease, modified diets should be available.

### Possible Nutritional Deficiencies in Adolescence

There are nutrients that may be lacking or low in some adolescent's diets. This occurs either because the nutrient content of the food is assumed rather than known, or because adolescents' diets have been shown to be low or deficient in foods that contain these nutrients. Also, there are some nutrients whose importance in growth has only recently been emphasized.

### Calcium and Vitamin D

Calcium requirements in adolescence are greater at the time of the growth spurt because of rapid skeletal growth. Vitamin D is needed to aid in the absorption of calcium. Both of these required nutrients can be obtained easily if adequate amounts of milk and milk products are consumed, provided that the milk and milk products are fortified with vitamin D.

Recommended calcium intakes are much higher than actual needs for growth, because an individual's absorptive efficiency may be very poor.

## Iron

The rapid growth in adolescence is also associated with an increased need for iron. Iron deficiency of concern in adolescence because studies indicate that adolescents may not ingest adequate iron for normal and increased needs during growth (Huenemann et al, 1974). It has been found that hematocrit for boys rises rapidly with increasing SMR, while that of the girls does not (Daniel, 1975). This is thought to be related to male testosterone production, which stimulates increased hemoglobin and erythrocyte production to nourish the rapidly growing muscle mass. Still, in the latter stages of growth, as girls begin to menstruate, their iron needs will be greater because of the iron loss.

Recommended intakes must be high because only a small percentage of ingested iron is absorbed. Intakes are limited because sources are limited and may be expensive. Therefore, adolescents are at risk for poor iron status and must be carefully assessed for iron intake.

The differential diagnosis of iron deficiency anemia is important as it may result from many causes. It can result from inadequate intakes of iron over a period of time. Iron deficiency anemia is most commonly diagnosed by determining hematocrit and hemoglobin. However, because hematological values are age and sex related, it is best when possible to obtain more information about iron stores. Serum iron and total iron-binding capacity can be used to estimate the percentage of transferrin saturation, indicative of body iron stores. Transferrin saturation of 16% or less is indicative of deficient body iron stores, and a value of less than 20%, is inadequate for boys (Daniel, 1975).

To obtain an indication of iron status, it is best to examine food intake information supplied by the individual or his parent or caregiver, or to examine menus for adequacy of iron sources. The best sources of iron are organ meats such as liver, closely followed by beef, chicken, veal, and fish, as well as soybeans. Iron found in animal products is better assimilated by the human body than foods of vegetable origin because of the form of the iron in the food. Other enhancing factors such as the amino acid content of the animal products, versus that of vegetable foods as a whole, appear to increase absorption of iron. Also, in the "typical" meal containing both animal and vegetable products, the total iron absorbed is greater than if there were only a single source. Further, even though products in this country like wheat, flour, and rice are fortified with iron, the amount of iron absorbed from these products is variable. The diet should include good sources of iron daily if possible, but at least several times weekly to assure optimal iron status.

**Other Nutrients to Consider**

Not all nutrients can be included in this discussion, but some deserve mention either because recent studies have brought attention to their importance or because of their possible lack in adolescents' diets.

Folic acid is essential during growth because it is needed for the synthesis of DNA and therefore is required for cell replication. It is highly interrelated with vitamin B12 and it is very difficult in some cases to distinguish between a deficiency of folic acid and vitamin B12. Diet information is very helpful because folic acid occurs in foods very different from those containing vitamin B12. During adolescence, folic acid may not be ingested in adequate amounts if the individual does not eat adequate amounts of fruits and vegetables.

Ascorbic acid has been found to be low in some adolescents' diets (Huenemann et al, 1974), when the adolescent does not consume citrus fruits and juices.

Vitamin A has been found to be low in some adolescents' diets (Huenemann et al, 1974). This is possible when intake of yellow fruits and vegetables is low and/or intake of whole milk or whole milk products is limited.

It has been found that the retention of zinc increases greatly at adolescence. If dietary zinc is not adequate at the time of onset of puberty, growth failure and delayed sexual maturation may occur. Zinc is found primarily in bone, but also in soft tissue. Because zinc is widely distributed in foods, deficiency is not normally a problem. However, deficiencies have been found to occur in areas of the world where excessive consumption of cereal containing large amounts of phytates inhibits iron and zinc absorption. Other factors affect zinc status, such as prolonged malabsorption and chronic infection.

**Nutrient Requirements Translated into Food Needs in Adolescence**

Very simply, one must consider foods served to and/or consumed by the adolescent in terms of quantity and quality. It has been pointed out that the quantity of food eaten in adolescence must be great because of needs for maintenance and activity as well as growth. In general, studies have shown that most adolescents consume adequate calories and protein. Still, this must be assured, and therefore, one must carefully monitor growth by plotting increments in height and weight, preferably on a standardized growth chart.

The quality of the diet is a different matter. It has already been pointed out that it may not be easy to consume adequate amounts of certain nutrients due to budget restraints and high growth requirements. However, it is also becoming clearer that some adolescents have very different eating patterns. Whether due to a desire to assert their independence, or peer pressure, these patterns must be acknowledged. It is important to recognize the diet as a whole and the contribution of foods eaten to overall nutrient needs. Huenemann et al (1974) found in their study of teenagers that for some, there was a tendency for snacking to replace meal eating, that some teens ate unusual foods for meals, and that obese subjects reported eating fewer meals and snacks than other subjects. Again, these practices are not necessarily harmful and may be very difficult to change.

The following are some very general guidelines for assuring adequate nutrient intake in adolescence:

1.  It is best to work with an individual's present diet. Try to overcome biases that affect judgment of someone else's habits. The focus should be on the quality and quantity of the nutrients in the diet as a whole.
2.  In meal planning or in evaluating an individual's intake, realize that growth demands are great, and that in order to get needed nutrients, high calorie foods with few or no nutrients must be kept to a minimum.
3.  Evaluate iron sources for the quality and quantity in the diet. Good sources of iron should be included at least several times a week.
4.  Evaluate fruit and vegetable intake for adequate folic acid, ascorbic acid, and vitamin A intake. Individuals should be encouraged to include fruits and vegetables as desserts and snacks.

5. Evaluate bulk in the diet to avoid or alleviate constipation problems. Cereal products such as bran, fruits, vegetables, and nuts
provide roughage needed to avoid or alleviate constipation. Fruit
juices are also helpful because they increase the moisture content
of excreta.
6. Evaluate the diet for milk and milk product content to assure adequate calcium and vitamin D intake. Further, one should not
assume that the milk contains adequate vitamin D. Most commercial milk is fortified to a specific, adequate level of vitamin D,
but local farm milk may not be.
7. Priorities should be set for improvement of diets. That is, when
the diet is inadequate in several ways, one cannot expect all
needed changes to be made at once.

**Factors Affecting the Nutritional**
**Requirements of Developmentally Disabled Adolescents**

Many factors that affect nutrient requirements of all adolescents have
already been discussed. Briefly, nutrient requirements vary between
boys and girls, according to developmental age, body size, activity,
and reproductive needs.

Of these factors, one that may affect more developmentally disabled adolescents than it does typical adolescents is activity. Some
severely physically disabled adolescents will have a tendency to
become obese because of inactivity. It is best to prevent the obesity by
assuring appropriate nutrient intake, and if possible some physical
activity. However, if obesity has developed, these adolescents should
be treated in the same manner as other obese adolescents, as described
earlier.

Another environmental factor to consider that may be more commonly found among these adolescents is emotional stress. Nutrient
requirements and energy metabolism can be altered by emotional
stress. Initially, the "stress" reaction may cause a release of glucose
into the bloodstream, but as glycogen stores (storage form of glucose)
are depleted, amino acids will be used for energy (Scrimshaw, 1969).
This release of energy sources is believed to occur because, in prehis-
toric man, stress reactions occurred to prepare the person for great
physical exertion. Protein may be diverted from its primary function
of tissue building when this reaction occurs. Other nutrients that are
affected include calcium, vitamin A, ascorbic acid, the B-complex
vitamins, and iron. Other nutritional effects are loss of appetite and a
tendency to change normal eating patterns. What this may mean in
terms of extra requirements for these nutrients depends on the nutri-

tional status of the individual, and the frequency, intensity, and duration of the stress.

## Developmentally Disabled Adolescents
## May Have Difficulty in Obtaining Adequate Nutrition

Some developmentally disabled adolescents will vary from other adolescents in their ability to obtain adequate nutrition. Most will have less cognitive ability and therefore, somewhat less ability to understand their nutritional needs. However, with appropriate nutrition education most mildly mentally handicapped adolescents should be able to understand their needs and how to meet them. Other, more mentally handicapped individuals may not be able to understand nutritional needs but can still be influenced to make wise food choices through parent or staff example and positive experiences with nutritious foods.

For many developmentally disabled adolescents, food served at home will be a strong force in forming food habits. Further, parent or staff attitudes toward food and examples that are set by these people are very important. Meals should be planned and food carefully purchased, prepared and stored, to assure adequate nutrient contents. Menus and food service should be planned or at least checked by a dietitian or nurse in the institution or group home. Further, attitudes of the parents toward feeding children should be explored in the home setting. Some parents use food inappropriately as a reward or may tend to overfeed as an expression of love.

Another environmental factor that may greatly affect both the adolescent's food intake and activity is his exposure to television and other forms of media. First, the adolescent is influenced by the food choices of those seen in commercials and food ads. Only about 3% of food advertising on television concerns nutritious food (Barcus, 1975). There is, rather, an overabundance of sweet and low nutritive foods. Further, the manner of presentation is one of demand rather than suggestion. Exactly how this affects the developmentally disabled adolescent is unknown. Still, one should consider how much time the adolescent spends watching television. Excessive television watching distracts from other activities and is a poor influence on wise food choice.

## Summary: Assessment of Nutritional Status

It seems best to summarize this section by offering an approach to the assessment of nutritional status and needs in developmentally disabled adolescents. Various levels of assessment are possible, depending on the facilities available, staff, access to a laboratory, time, and funds. Further, the type of assessment depends on the purpose of the evaluation.

Every clinic, institution, group home, or school must take some responsibility for determining nutritional status of their adolescents. Table 2 contains suggested approaches and procedures based on the extent of the assessment desired and the limitations of the setting. Some aspects of these assessments deserve further discussion.

*Dietary Evaluation*    There are many ways to assess food and nutrient intake, but not all of these are practical with developmentally disabled adolescents. The method chosen should depend on whether an individual or group is being evaluated, the individual's cognitive level and/or parents' ability to provide information, the purpose of obtaining the information, time and staff limitations.

A check for adequacy in the "Basic Four Food Groups" (U.S.D.A., 1958) gives an indication of the quality of an individual's diet. This is practical for checking institutional or group home food service and for recall by some individual adolescents. It can involve a check of the foods eaten the day before or a check of the usual pattern. Obviously, the information obtained is not very specific or accurate.

A recall of foods eaten, in specific amounts, on the day before (24-hour food recall), is a commonly used method that can determine fairly accurately quality and quantity of intake. It can be used in the clinical setting and possibly in other settings. This information must be obtained from parents or caregivers. It suffers from the fact that it is indicative of only one day. An idea of how typical the intake was should be obtained by asking the adolescent's parent. One should try to obtain some information from the adolescent. Some can recall the last meal eaten. This is important not for food intake information, but for food awareness information. The adolescent may have no awareness of foods eaten and this may be part of the need in a nutrition education program.

If time permits, in the institution and some group homes, a very accurate method of assessing food intake is to observe food intake for a day or on several days. This would not be practical in settings where the adolescents do not have at least two meals to be observed. One should ask the adolescent if he or she ate anything else beyond what was recorded.

The 3- to 7-day food records provide accurate indications of food and nutrient intake, but for most efficient use these methods require that the person using the information obtained know how to determine nutrient content and compare results to standards. Nutrient contents of foods can be obtained from several publications including, *Food Values of Portions Commonly Used* (Church and Church, 1975).

When asking the adolescent or parent about intake, avoid suggesting meals or snacks. For example, instead of asking whether or not the adolescent had breakfast, ask when and what was first eaten at the beginning of the day. Further, attempt to get full information about foods, such as serving size and method of preparation (quantitative methods only). Also, one should ask about food supplements such as vitamins and minerals.

*Clinical Evaluation*   Every adolescent's height and weight should be monitored. It is best to plot these measures on a standardized growth chart such as the Tanner, National Child Health Survey, or Stuart grids.

The individual should be measured with a stable, nonflexible tape or board without shoes and with his body fully extended. Weight should be determined on a balance type scale without shoes and extra clothing.

The most accurate growth information is obtained over time. That is, one measure gives an indication of present status, but is not nearly as accurate as several measures over a period of time. The individual's normal growth channel on a standardized chart is best seen with several measures and is a better indicator of growth and nutritional needs.

*Laboratory Evaluation*   Biochemical or laboratory evaluation is probably only practical in the clinical and community settings. When this kind of evaluation is possible, a determination should be made of the levels of blood forming nutrients: iron, folic acid, vitamin B6, and vitamin B12. The most common laboratory assessments are hematocrit and hemoglobin. Whenever iron status is questionable, iron stores should be evaluated by measuring serum iron and total iron-binding capacity, and determining transferrin saturation. Values should be correlated to sexual maturity and stage of growth.

## NUTRITION EDUCATION

The definition of nutrition education implies a process whereby diet changes occur through changes in knowledge and attitudes. Nutrition education may involve one person or many people. In the clinical and home settings, the process usually involves the educator and one

Table 2.    Assessment of nutritional status of adolescents

| Level | Dietary | Clinical | Laboratory |
|---|---|---|---|
| I (minimum level for clinical, home, group home, institution) | Qualitative information: <br> 1. Frequency of use of "Basic Four Food Groups" (U.S.D.A., 1958) <br> 2. Eating patterns: meals, snacks <br><br> Clinical, home: <br> 3. From parents: amount spent on groceries weekly; use of food stamps; eligibility for aid. <br><br> Group home, institution: <br> 3. Food service evaluation: meal planning, adequacy in food groups, quality in storage, preparation, serving. | 1. Height <br> 2. Weight (plot on standardized growth chart; follow over time.) <br> 3. External appearance | Clinical, other settings whenever possible: <br> 1. Hematocrit <br> 2. Hemoglobin |

| | | |
|---|---|---|
| II | Above plus 1. Quantitative information: 24-hour recall on foods eaten<br><br>Group home, institution: 2. Observe foods eaten for 1 day | Above plus Clinical: 1. For those suspected to be obese or overweight: arm circumference skinfold thickness | Above plus Clinical: 1. For those suspected to have poor iron status: serum iron,[a] total iron-binding capacity[a] |
| III | Above plus 1. Quantitative information: 3–7 day food record | | Above plus 1. Blood: vitamin A, beta carotene, cholesterol, zinc, folic acid 2. Urine: zinc, thiamine, riboflavin, protein, sugar 3. Hair shaft analysis for protein, zinc, other metals[b] |

Adapted from: Christakis, George, 1973. Nutritional assessment in health programs. Am. J. Pub. Health 63:55.

[a] Per standards found in: Daniel, W. A., Gaines, E. G., and Bennett, D. L. 1975. Iron intake and transferrin saturation in adolescents. J. Pediatr. 86:288–292.

[b] For further information: Heald, F. P., 1976. New reference points for defining adolescent nutrient requirements. In J. I. McKigney and H. N. Munro (eds.), Nutrient Requirements in Adolescence. MIT Press, Cambridge, Mass.

person or one family. In the institutional or group home setting the education may involve one person, but will usually involve more. Still it is important to consider "individuals" as often as possible, even the individuals in a group, because each will be affected by different cognitive, social, and environmental factors.

As an educational process, nutrition education involves various methods, techniques, procedures, and illustrative materials to inform and influence food practices (Todhunter, 1969). One must be careful to choose these according to the cognitive and social abilities of the individual or group. The process begins very simply with posters and photographs placed in the environment, to create interest. The process then continues in steps building greater understanding and acceptance of nutrition.

Nutrition education effectiveness may be evaluated by some in terms of immediate changes in diet or growth. The best evaluation focuses on very small changes, starting with knowledge or attitude. These small changes add up in the long run and are more effective than sudden drastic changes.

The need for nutrition education may be based on the assessment of an individual's or group's nutritional status and/or a desire for these adolescents to live independently and successfully as adults. Even for those who will never live independently, many will still have some degree of control over their intake and should be educated to make wise food choices. In institutions or group homes, it is not enough to provide nutritious food. In group homes where individuals are prepared for independent living, it is also not enough to teach basic cooking skills.

It is important for as many of these adolescents as possible to learn to take responsibility for their own food intake. However, they may lack basic motivation to learn about foods and nutrition. For example, there is evidence that nutrition is not a popular subject in public schools. That nutrition is dull and boring is a common opinion of teachers and administrators, as well as students. Some feel that students do not apply what they learn about nutrition anyway, so why bother? Still, these educators and students desire that each student be able to get a job and adjust successfully in an independent living situation as an adult. This clearly requires that the individual have a basis and motivation to choose nutritious foods that will promote optimal health. Further, it has been found that when it is presented in an interesting and personal manner, nutrition education has been successful.

## General Guidelines for the Assessment
## and Planning of Nutrition Education Needs

Whether in a clinical, institutional, group home, or school setting, some general guidelines should be followed in assessing and planning for nutrition education needs. Accompanying these guidelines, is a study conducted by this author that attempted to assess nutrition education needs among mildly mentally handicapped adolescents in the public schools and emotionally disturbed adolescents in a group home setting. While the public school is probably an ideal setting for nutrition education, some valuable insight on needs assessment in other settings can still be gained from the study.

*Determine the Priority Individuals or Groups in Need of Nutrition Education*   In any setting, one must first consider who has control over the food service. That is, appropriate, nutritious foods should be served to the individual or group of adolescents as the primary influence over food intake. In institutions or group homes, one should consider the food service and cooks. In the home setting, the parent may be or may not be providing most of the adolescent's food. Some of these adolescents may live on their own and take care of all of their own food needs. In the home setting, the adolescent and his parent can usually be educated together, if foods available are inappropriate. In the institution or group home, however, inappropriate food service is more difficult to deal with.

If it is found in the institutional or group home setting that there is need for nutrition education of the food service and house staff, one should seek the assistance of a registered dietitian or nutritionist. Most state health departments have a nutritionist available for consultation to institutions. Only a few will have a nutritionist available for consultation to group homes. However, there are usually consulting nutritionists in the community who can be hired.

Most adolescents have some control over their own food intake. After considering foods served in the home, institution, or group home, then the adolescent should be assessed for nutrition education needs in terms of his ability and desire to utilize food resources presently and in the future.

*Determine the Nutrition Education Needs of the Target Group or Individual*   A study of "the nutrition information, attitudes, and practices of mildly mentally retarded adolescents" (Greenwood, 1977) was conducted to determine the nutrition education needs of this population in a public school system. Some information was also obtained concerning the needs of emotionally disturbed adolescents in a group home setting. This study can be used as an example of how needs could be assessed. Thirty public school subjects and eight group home subjects were interviewed by means of an orally administered questionnaire of approximately 40 minutes duration. Questions were of several types: open-ended, information seeking questions were the most frequent type, agree or disagree questions were asked to ascertain more information and attitudes and opinion questions were asked as indicators of attitudes and practices. Last meal recall was used as an indication of food awareness. Cards with pictures of foods (National Dairy Council. 1974. Chicago, Ill.) were used as aids for food identification. For other questions, real photographs of objects or people or depicting a scene were used to aid the adolescent in understanding the question (Figure 1).

In general, the adolescents seemed to enjoy answering the questions and answered them freely. The questions answered most appropriately appeared to be those involving concrete concepts, familiar things or experiences, and those concerning cooking.

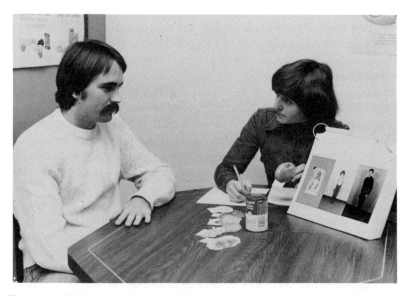

Figure 1. Visual aids used in a study (Greenwood, 1977) to help mildly mentally retarded adolescents understand and answer questions more fully. The foods cards (National Dairy Council, 1974, Chicago, Ill.) were used for food identification, source, and content questions. The can of soup was used in a cooking question. The poster boards with photographs were used for many types of questions.

In assessing needs, it is most important to begin with the simplest concepts. One should first consider food awareness. In the public school study (Greenwood, 1977) the adolescent was shown ten food items and asked what they were. All foods were named correctly by most except two. This was most likely due to the quality of those two food pictures, but was also due to unfamiliarity with the two items.

When asked what was in the food or where the food came from, more had difficulty in answering. Only between 50 and 67% could correctly identify the source or content of the foods shown to them. This points to a need to teach about foods and the food supply as well as about food as it is needed for health and growth.

About 25% gave a correctly named nutrient in the food as an answer to this question concerning food content. However, it was later shown in two different types of questions that their knowledge was lacking because many incorrect nutrient responses concerning the same foods were given. For example, even though in the first question about 25% said oranges have vitamin C in them, in a later opinion question, 87% thought fruits have a lot of protein in them. This is not to say that they know nothing of nutrient content, but that they may be parotting answers and may not really understand nutrients and their importance. "Nutrients" is an abstract concept, and it may be that some will never understand it and should not be confused by including such concepts in their curriculum.

After basic food awareness, source and content, the questions began to explore their understanding of nutrition in relation to health and growth. When asked why we eat foods, 70% had a general answer such as "for health" or "for growth." Concerning growth, each adolescent was shown a series of three pictures: baby, 3-year-old boy, and teenage boy, and asked to describe what happened when a person went from "here" (baby) to "here" (adolescent). Almost all (92%) mentioned growth. When asked about appropriate foods for the baby, 89% were able to mention at least one appropriate food. When asked whether the little boy would eat different foods than the baby, 68% thought he would, and of these, 50% said he would eat more. The other 18% did not know what would be different. Discussion of and knowledge of needs at different life stages is especially important for adolescents who are preparing for independent living.

Questions dealing with awareness of growth measures and appropriate ways to lose weight showed these adolescents to be very aware of scales and height measures and appropriate ways to lose weight. However, when questioned about personal experience with attempts to lose weight, many more inappropriate methods were mentioned. This points to the need to involve the adolescent to a greater extent in the learning process and to consider ways to motivate the adolescent to apply what he learns.

The questions then moved into the areas of meal planning, food purchasing, and awareness of community resources for food and other needs. Based on author opinion, 44% were able to choose balanced meals, while 56% did not. It was also found that 88% had shopped before, but of these, only 41% had shopped alone. Community resource awareness revealed some interesting results. The adolescent was asked where he would go if he were living alone and had run out of money for food. About 25% could name two resources and 25% one resource. The other 50% could not think of any community resources that would help them. It was probably the case that those who knew of resources had had experience with this in their own families. In any case, this emphasizes the need to increase awareness among those who are preparing for independent living.

The final area explored concerned cooking and safety skills. Most adolescents demonstrated cooking experience and knew appropriate safety measures.

Many other types of assessment are possible. To obtain more information about food awareness, one can observe food choices or ask the adolescent at several visits what he or she had to eat at the last meal. The adolescent could also demonstrate food purchasing, preparing, and storing skills. Whatever method is used, it is most important to assess knowledge and skill levels as soon as possible and begin assessment at a basic level. A copy of the final questionnaire developed to assess the nutrition information attitudes, and practices of mildly mentally handicapped adolescents can be obtained by writing to the author.

Studying the needs of mildly mentally handicapped adolescents resulted in the following recommendations.

1. More careful planning of the food and nutrition curriculum in home economics in this public school setting was needed. The curriculum should be based on assessment of needs and planned with objectives, methods, and activities for each nutrition concept.
2. Basic nutrition and food preparation should be taught concomitantly, not separately as currently done. Actually, food preparation should be the learning activity used to reinforce food and nutrition concepts.
3. How to shop and use public assistance agencies should be taught

and reinforced with visits and experience in these community settings.

In other settings, one should have access to more background information on each adolescent than was available for this study. Information on past experience in food and nutrition classes, as well as family history of socioeconomic status and disease should be utilized to aid in planning nutrition education for these adolescents.

*Know the Abilities of the Group or Individual*  Beyond determining needs, before really beginning to plan nutrition education, one must know the abilities of the group or individual. First, this refers to the cognitive abilities. Very often, one will be very familiar with the cognitive level of the individual or group, but if not, this should be determined. One may have to deal with many levels of cognition at once. In the group home setting, for example, there may be mildly and moderately handicapped individuals. One should begin at the lowest level, but offer more advanced information to those interested and capable.

Most important, one should not assume that the individual or group has a good understanding of foods and nutrition merely because he claims to have such understanding. Whenever possible, demonstration of knowledge is best. This is especially important if cooking will be included in the education. To do this, one might, for example, begin by having the individual or group prepare a food or dish. One can observe safety skills and proper cooking procedure. Further, one can get an indication of the social adjustment of various members of the group.

Nutrition education, then, should be planned according to cognitive and social levels, as well as cooking safety and skills. This should include all aspects of the education, from posters to materials and approach. Further, it happens all too often that the level of education is too high because the educator is overly concerned about making nutrition interesting. One should devise objectives, steps, and methods, and assure that the individual or group is comfortable with each step before continuing. For some moderately retarded individuals, it will take months to understand what food is made of, and why it is important to eat certain foods. Appropriate creativity can certainly help to deter boredom and enhance learning over the necessary time period.

*Fit the Education into Existing Values and Patterns*  It is most important to determine present eating practices when improvement or change is desired. In considering changes needed, one or two should be chosen with or for the individual or group to work on. One must be very careful to consider the quality and quantity of foods eaten as a whole and avoid personal bias. Further, familiarity with various cultural food patterns helps. Nutrition education is most effective when the educator begins with what the individual or group is presently consuming and makes only small changes.

Further, one should avoid biases about meals and snacks. Again, the overall quality and quantity must be examined. Also, dislikes and likes are held by most people and these should be respected. Developmentally disabled adolescents may display some unusual food behaviors that for the most part should be ignored. For example, some may have food jags left over from childhood that serve as attention getting devices.

Some food behaviors may not be acceptable or may become exaggerated, requiring intervention. Eating appropriately is a cognitive function and for some may have to be learned. In some individuals, inappropriate behaviors may lead to a grossly inadequate diet that can affect growth and health. When behavior is unacceptable or the individual's growth or health is at stake, further evaluation by a behavior therapist and nutritionist is needed.

For most individuals, however, small diet changes will be adequate and group education feasible. One can determine something about present food patterns by several methods, as described earlier. (See "Dietary Evaluation" in the nutritional requirements section.) It is important to remember that even though the adolescent may not be able to provide accurate food intake information, this information usually can be obtained in another way. What is important is questioning the adolescent about his intake to determine food awareness.

**Environmental Factors to Consider**   It is most important to assess what strengths and limitations individual adolescents or groups of adolescents have in various settings. Some of the present limitations may require change before a nutrition education program can begin.

Has nutrition education ever been part of the clinical, community, institutional, or group home setting? In most cases, the idea will never have been considered and there may not be awareness of its importance. The nurse may have to create in the staff an awareness of its importance and its benefits to developmentally disabled adolescents. In many group living situations, where residents are preparing for independent living, food preparation, storage, and serving may be taught. However, this is not nutrition education; it will not necessarily cause improvement or establishment of proper eating habits. Further, this does not relate to individual nutritional needs and possible future family needs. Evidence that food preparation, storage, and serving are not nutrition education often comes when, after the individual has left and established independent living, he cooks T.V. dinners every night! This occurs because the individual had nothing to base food choices on and/or because he was not motivated to improve eating habits. Nutrition concepts and education activities like cooking should be taught concomitantly. All too often, high school home economics teachers plan a "nutrition" unit for 1 week and a "cooking" unit for at least 6 weeks! The two should not be separated in mind or practice. In other settings, the nurse should institute changes in the process of nutrition education by pointing out the importance of proper nutrition education based on principles of nourishment, not cooking techniques. Further, effectiveness should be demonstrated through a carefully planned pilot study.

Another environmental consideration is the amount and type of activity the individual or group receives. One should consider whether or not time is allotted for physical activity, and what facilities and equipment are available. A part of this is considering how much time is spent watching television. An uncontrolled television in an environment may be overused. Some of the television time could be replaced with other activities. Physical activity should be regularly scheduled in institutions and group homes as well as in the home setting.

A third consideration are the facilities and equipment available for resident or individual participation in cooking or serving as a nutrition education activity. In the clinical setting there may or may not be cooking facilities. Still, for occasional food demonstrations, one could use any room with a table, bringing equipment from home and preparing foods that do not have to be cooked. In the institution or group home, the problem may be access to the kitchen and cooking facilities. Many places, though, will already have the adolescents involved at least in serving food already prepared. Possibly other special arrangements for food demonstrations could be made.

One should also consider the community as a whole. There are learning laboratories in most facilities that, if tapped, could be valuable and enjoyable nutrition education tools. Shopping trips can both promote better food choices and teach individuals how to shop. These are a must for adolescents preparing for independent living. In working with physically handicapped individuals, showing them how they can shop will build their confidence and increase the likelihood of their shopping alone in the future. There may also be farms, bakeries, and food processing plants where field trips could be taken. There are still many mentally handicapped adolescents who have never been told about or shown how foods are grown or raised and how they reach the market.

*Determine All Possible Avenues for Nutrition Education*    After an environmental assessment, consider all resources at hand that could be used to teach nutrition to the target individual or group. This includes materials in the environment, materials that can be obtained free or within a budget, and people in the setting or community.

Nutrition education can be taught and learned passively or actively. When time is heavily limited, posters, photographs, and displays in the environment can be a form of nutrition education. These serve as models to the individual or group. If chosen carefully they stimulate interest. They may raise questions from viewers and stimulate further planning.

Also passively, the staff must serve as models. This cannot be overstressed in the institutional, group home, or school setting. It is pointless to plan nutrition education if the opposite example is practiced by the staff. This is not to say that one must give up all low nutritive foods at all times to teach nutrition education. Rather, if one professes that balanced meals are important, for example, eating a candy bar for lunch would cancel the effectiveness of the education (Figure 2).

Actively, the possibilities are endless. Many were alluded to in considering environmental factors. These were cooking, field trips, and shopping trips. Generally an individual or group progresses from little or no personal involvement to greater and greater involvement. Again, the extent of the program will be determined by time and staff available. However, one will find that if community resources are sought out, assistance can be found.

**Specific Nutrition Education Suggestions**

Table 3 summarizes the possibilities for nutrition education in various settings. Level I contains simple educational procedures that are passive or that do not directly involve the adolescents themselves. These methods are especially effective in creating interest in nutrition, but have limited effectiveness in promoting learning. The best way to enhance learning is to involve the adolescent directly as suggested in levels II and III. This is by no means a complete list of suggestions, and it is hoped that other will be created and/or utilized in various settings. Some aspects of the table deserve further comment.

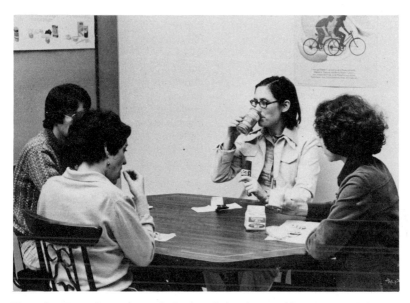

Figure 2.   Poor educator example (center of photo) at mealtime can cancel the effectiveness of the whole nutrition education program, no matter how well planned and extensive it may be.

***Photographs, Posters, and Displays***   Whenever possible, real pictures of real persons and objects should be used as visual aids. Developmentally disabled adolescents need a clear understanding of the message and this is best obtained by using real photographs. Further, when possible, pictures of the adolescents themselves participating in a nutrition education activity should be used.

Posters and displays are effective too, especially when they are colorful and unusual (Figure 3). These should be placed discretely in the environment. As "active" nutrition education, some students can help make posters and displays.

The photographs or posters can depict many things. Nutritious foods shown in attractive ways and people enjoying nutritious foods will serve as an influence to make nutritious food choices. The source of foods can also be depicted. For example, a series of pictures could depict how grain becomes bread. The importance of good nutrition for growth and health is more difficult to show, but there are ways to do it. The relationship could be suggested by combining pictures of nutritious foods and adolescents participating in various physical activities on the same poster. Finally, different nutrition education

Table 3. Nutrition education in various settings

| Level | Clinical/community | Home | Institution/group home |
|---|---|---|---|
| Level I | 1. Posters Photographs Displays<br>2. Discussion with individual about growth, diet, activity needs Growth charts Food cards Food models Physical activity charts | 1. Posters Photographs<br>2. Same as clinical/community<br>3. Parent modeling; availability of nutritious, tasty food | 1. Posters Photographs Displays<br>2. Same as clinical/community<br>3. Staff modeling; availability of nutritious tasty food |
| Level II | Above plus<br>1. Food demonstration —cooking, tasting<br>2. Help adolescent learn to weigh and measure himself<br>3. Plan activities with adolescent and parent<br>4. Plan shopping trips | Above plus<br>1. Meal planning, budgeting, and use of recipes with parent<br>2. Encourage adolescent participation in meal planning, purchasing and preparation<br>3. Plan activities with adolescent and parent | Above plus<br>1. Place food games in environment<br>2. Tour kitchen of institution<br>3. Work with individual adolescent on food intake<br>4. Assure adequate activity programs<br>5. Plan shopping trips; trips to community agencies like the food stamp office |
| Level III | Above plus<br>1. Growth demonstrations plants, animals (Martin, 1963)<br>2. Adolescent could plan, purchase, and prepare simple foods | 1. Same as clinical/community | 1. Same as clinical/community<br>2. Hold group discussions and activities; plan objectives, methods, materials, activities<br>3. Involve adolescent in food preparation, storage, service when possible (see text) |

activities can be encouraged by displaying pictures of some adolescents enjoying an activity. For example, pictures of the teens enjoying a field trip or shopping trip could be displayed.

***Planning Activities for "Active" Nutrition Education***    In levels II and II (Table 3), as the nutrition education process becomes more involved, one should carefully plan goals, objectives, and methods for adolescent education to assure that appropriate learning occurs. Concepts should proceed as suggested earlier in needs assessment, that is, from food and its content and source, to food and its importance in growth and health, including how to plan and prepare food to meet growth and health needs. Other concepts that could be included, beyond the two basic ones suggested, might be foods of different cultures or how food is used to entertain. There are many possibilities, but it is suggested that the adolescent have a solid understanding of the basic concepts before proceeding to others. For most developmentally disabled adolescents, nutrients should not be discussed. Rather, foods in general should be the focus. Also, small steps may have to be planned for some adolescents. Again, through assessment of food knowledge and skills, one will have the best idea of needs and where to begin.

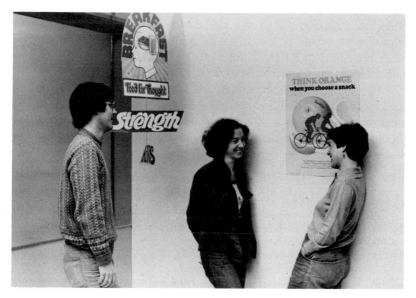

Figure 3.   Multicolored and shaped posters can be very effective tools in creating interest in nutrition and promoting improvement of eating habits.

*Considerations in Adolescent Cooking Experiences*   It must again be emphasized that cooking experiences should be related to certain food concepts, as learning activities. Also, it is most important to carefully assess food preparation, storage, and safety skills before beginning a program. There will be some adolescents who cannot open a can and others who can cook complex dishes. Further, some adolescents are unsafe in the kitchen and this must be discovered as well.

Overall, instituting a successful cooking program requires familiarity with many home economics principles. For the nurse in most settings, one-to-one cooking activities, possibly with some consultation from an experienced home economist, are best.

*Resources*   Assistance in planning and developing a nutrition education program is not widely available. There may be a home economist or nutritionist in the community that could be hired as a private consultant. If one is fortunate enough to be near a community or state college or university one could consult the home economics department. Planning nutrition education for developmentally disabled adolescents or assisting in the planning would be a good student project.

Individual adolescents and their families may be able to receive assistance from a government program. The Expanded Food and Nutrition Program will accept referrals of families who meet certain requirements, such as low socioeconomic status. There may also be other programs in different areas. One should check the local extension office of the United States Department of Agriculture.

For materials, local sources are available in most areas. Many food producers distribute nutrition information materials, such as local dairy farmers or fruit and vegetable growers. Government offices should be checked, such as the local extension office of the United States Department of Agriculture and the Federal Government Printing Office (local branch).

## REFERENCES CITED

Barcus, F. E. 1975a. Television in the After School Hours. Action for Children's Television, Newtonville, Mass.

Barcus, F. E. 1975b. Weekend Commercial Children's Television. Action for Children's Television, Newtonville, Mass.

Church, C. F. and Church, H. N. 1975. Food Values of Portions Commonly Used. 12th ed. J. P. Lippincott, Philadelphia.

Cooke, R. E. 1969. The basic principles of energy balance. In: F. P. Heald (ed.), Adolescent Nutrition and Growth. Appleton-Century-Crofts, New York.

Daniel, W. A., Gaines, E. G., and Bennett, D. L. 1975. Iron intake and transferrin saturation in adolescents. J. Pediatr. 86:288–292.

Garn, S. M., and Wagner, B. 1969. The adolescent growth of the skeletal mass and its implications to mineral requirements. In: F. P. Heald (ed.), Adolescent Nutrition and Growth, p. 140. Appleton-Century-Crofts, New York.

Greenwood, M. H. 1977. Survey of: The nutrition information, attitudes, and practices of mildly mentally retarded adolescents. Unpublished master's thesis, University of Washington.

Heald, F. P. (ed.). 1969. Adolescent Nutrition and Growth. Appleton-Century-Crofts, New York.

Heald, F. P., Mayer, J., and Remmell, P. S. 1969. Calorie, protein, and fat intakes in children. In: F. P. Heald (ed.), Adolescent Nutrition and Growth. Appleton-Century-Crofts, New York.

Hegsted, D. M. 1976. Current knowledge of energy, fat, protein, and amino acid needs of adolescents. In: J. I. McKigney and H. N. Munro (eds.), Nutrient Requirements in Adolescence, pp. 114 and 119. MIT Press, Cambridge, Mass

Huenemann, R. L., Hampton, M. C., Behnke, A. R., Shapiro, L. R., and Mitchell, B. W. 1974. Teenage Nutrition and Physique. Charles C Thomas, Springfield, Ill.

Johnston, J. A. 1958. Protein requirements of adolescents. Ann. N.Y. Acad. Sci. 69:881.

Martin, E. A. 1963. Nutrition Education in Action. Holt, Rinehart and Winston, New York.

Mayer, J. 1972. Human Nutrition: Its Physiological, Medical and Social Aspects. Charles C Thomas, Springfield, Ill.

McKigney, J. I., and Munro, H. N. 1976. Nutrient Requirements in Adolescence. MIT Press, Cambridge, Mass.

Scrimshaw, N. S. 1969. The effect of stress on nutrition in adolescents and young adults. In: F. P. Heald (ed.), Adolescent Nutrition and Growth. Appleton-Century-Crofts, New York.

Tanner, J. M. 1968. Growth at Adolescence. (2nd ed.). Blackwell Scientific, Oxford.

Todhunter, E. N. 1969. Approaches to nutrition education. J. Nutr. Educ. 1:8–9.

U.S.D.A. 1958. Food for Fitness: A Daily Food Guide. Leaflet No. 424.

## Sources for Standardized Growth Charts

National Center for Health Statistics. NCHS Growth Charts. 1976. Monthly Vital Statistics Report Vol. 25, No. 3, Supp. (HRA). 76–1120. Health Resources Administration, Rockville, Md.

Stuart, H. C. Anthropometric Chart. Copies can be obtained from Mead Johnson Laboratories.

Tanner, J. M., and Whitehouse, R. H. Growth and Development Record (Boys and Girls). Reference GDB11. University of London, Institute of Child Health, for the Hospital Sick Children, Great Ormond Street, London, W.C.1.

# chapter ten
# VOCATIONAL NEEDS

Kevin P. Lynch, Ph.D.

As a result of mandatory education acts, deinstitutionalization programs, the advocacy of parent groups, and decisions regarding the right to treatment within institutions (*Wyatt v. Aderholt*, 1971), we are now seeing a significant increase in the number of developmentally disabled children and adults who remain in the community. In many cities and towns these children and adolescents are being provided with preschool and school-age programs that should result in increases in their functioning level. While parents and professionals alike should continue to foster the development of quality training programs for school-age children, they should also be mindful of the need to ensure that their children's training is preparing them for life in the community. Naturally, for all of us, a very important aspect of our life in the community is our occupation. In the ethic of the western world, one's identity and status are in large measure determined by one's vocation. To the very great detriment of the developmentally disabled student, there exists no conceptual model for the vocational education and subsequent vocational placement of these citizens.

It is the intent of this chapter to provide the practitioner outside of the discipline of vocational education and vocational rehabilitation with an overview of current vocational programs for the developmentally disabled. To that end, selected research studies and a general overview of training methods will be discussed. The current status of vocational education and vocational rehabilitation programming will be explored and alternative models suggested. For an in-depth review of training and supervision procedures, the reader is referred to Bellamy (1976). For an overview of the broader issues of rehabilitation of the severely handicapped, the reader is referred to Gold (1973) and Wolfensberger (1967).

## THE PRODUCTIVE CAPACITY
## OF THE DEVELOPMENTALLY DISABLED

There continues to exist the widely held, yet generally erroneous notion, that the developmentally disabled cannot be taught to work. There are studies, however, which demonstrate conclusively that with the systematic application of specific procedures, it is possible to train developmentally disabled individuals to work successfully at tasks which might be considered complex in industrial settings. Loos and Tizard (1955) trained six "imbeciles" to fold and glue paper cake boxes. Clarke and Heremelin (1955) taught a similar group of people to sever electric wires to a specific length, to assemble nine component bicycle pumps, and to solder four color coded wires to a similar number of color coded terminals in an electronic assembly. More recently, Crosson (1966, 1969) trained seven severely retarded adults, whose mean IQ was 27, to complete a task requiring the use of a drill press in the manufacture of wood pencil holders, and a second task requiring the use of a hammer in assembling flower boxes. In the flower box assembly, the component parts of each task were analyzed and the assembly behaviors were modeled by the trainer. The subject was then prompted to imitate trainer behavior. Correct worker responses were reinforced with candy, praise, and tokens. The extrinsic reinforcers were faded over successive training trials.

Gold and associates (Gold, 1972, 1974; Gold and Barclay, 1973) have developed a training procedure which has proven to be effective in the assembly of a complex bicycle brake unit. In a one-to-one training situation, the client is seated before a partitioned training board that is sufficiently large (3 ft. × 1 ft.) to contain the 14 pieces of the Bendix RX 70 coaster brake assembly. The trainer sits next to the client and models strict attention to the task (e.g., the trainer does not maintain eye contact with the client), and subsequently models the entire assembly of the unit including the modeling of a correction procedure (e.g., the trainer purposely begins to make an assembly error and then states aloud "try another way" which he then corrects). After one modeling sequence, the client is trained over a series of trials until a specified criterion (six out of eight assemblies without errors or assistance) is met.

Bellamy, Peterson, and Close (1975) trained two profoundly retarded adults to assemble a 19-piece cam switch actuator. Following a task analysis of the assembly, the client was seated in front of a training board with the parts arranged in order. The assembly procedure was modeled by a trainer and the client was then required to imitate the assembly behavior. Correct responses were reinforced with consumables, praise, and physical contact. Incorrect responses were followed by a variety of correction procedures (p. 12) involving verbal directions, physical priming, and modeling. The client was then required to repeat the corrected step.

In a series of experiments conducted at the Vocational Services Component of the Institute for the Study of Mental Retardation and Related Disabilities at the University of Michigan, five moderately mentally retarded adults (average IQ, 51) with no previous work experience were taught the assembly of a 16-piece plastic flush valve which required, during the assembly process, the use of a pneumatic screwdriver. In the training procedure, the clients were desensitized to the high pitched whine and vibrations of the pneumatic screwdriver by the trainer, who modeled lack of fear in using the device. The trainer modeled the complete assembly of the flush valve and asked the client to imitate his behavior. Using these procedures, clients were able to approximate the productive capacity of sheltered workshop employees (a production rate of one-half the capacity of a nonhandicapped worker) during a 3-week training period.

As this evidence demonstrates, it is abundantly clear that developmentally disabled clients of varying functioning levels are capable of working successfully at comparatively complex tasks when systematic training procedures are employed.

## VOCATIONAL TRAINING PROCEDURES

In training the developmentally disabled worker, most successful studies have reported the use of modeling, shaping, physical priming, and verbal directions. However, before any training can commence with either a simple or complex assembly, it is imperative that the task be thoroughly analyzed by a process known as "task analysis." In analyzing a particular task, the elements of the assembly are examined to determine the most simple and economical procedures for assembly. The nature of the discriminations to be made for each element of the assembly is noted and, subsequently, a training procedure is devised that is based upon the needs of the individual client. As a result of task analysis and the devising of a training procedure, each client will be assured continuity of training method over many trials even if trainers are changed. Additionally, the presentation of the elements to the client will remain the same over many trials, thereby facilitating the client's discrimination learning.

## Shaping

In shaping, the client's initial gross and uneconomical overt responses to the stimulus features of the assembly are reinforced by the trainer. During each trial and through successive trials, however, the trainer reinforces narrower and more economical responses until the client reaches some agreed upon criterion level.

## Modeling

Modeling procedures employed in laboratory, clinical, institutional, and educational settings have consistently demonstrated to be effective and reliable with respect to a wide variety of teaching and/or training procedures (Bandura, 1969; Flanders, 1968). While many questions remain unanswered about the role of reinforcement and model status in imitation learning, there is general agreement that there is a phenomenon known as modeling and that under certain circumstances, subjects will imitate the actions of models, thereby acquiring whole chains of behavior economically. In a typical modeling paradigm, the model rehearses all of the behaviors associated with the assembly and then asks the client to reproduce the exact behavior. The client's reproduction of the model behavior is then reinforced. In a study comparing the relative effectiveness of low verbal training procedures, high verbal training procedures, and a reinforced video modeling procedure (Lynch and Malian, 1977) in teaching a 14-piece Bendix RX 70 coaster brake assembly to a population of severely and moderately retarded adults, it was found that the video modeling procedure trained clients to criterion significantly faster ($p < .001$) than either high verbal or low verbal methods employing priming, verbal labels, and shaping without video modeling.

## Physical Priming

In physical priming, the trainer physically moves the client through the correct motor responses associated with an element of the assembly task. In some cases, this may involve moving the client's hands through the motor manipulations associated with the task. Very severely involved clients may require extensive physical priming during training.

**Verbal Directions**

Providing the client with verbal directions and verbal cues has been shown to be an effective training device (Lynch and Malian, 1977; Gold and Barclay, 1973). Naturally, verbal cues and verbal directions are less effective when training clients with decreased levels of receptive language.

In the systematic application of modeling, physical priming, and the provision of verbal directions, the trainer attempts to shape client assembly behavior to reduce or eliminate the pauses and hesitations that are usually associated with learning new discriminations. While the trainer will initially provide the client with all necessary assistance, in the final analysis, the client should be able to perform the task at high levels of error-free production independent of the trainer. The process of gradually reducing the trainer involvement in shaping client behavior is "fading." In fading physical primes, for instance, the trainer may initially grasp the client's hands and move the hands through manipulations associated with an element of the assembly. On the next trial, the trainer may only grasp the client's wrist. Over subsequent trials, priming for that element may be reduced to a touch on the forearm, then just pointing to the correct bin, glancing at the right bin, until it is no longer necessary at all for the trainer to intervene as the client emits the correct response at the presentation of that stimulus.

It is abundantly clear that developmentally disabled workers are capable of productive enterprise and, as citizens, should be afforded access to training and, subsequently, the opportunity to be productive in the community.

## CURRENT STATUS OF VOCATIONAL EDUCATION
## AND VOCATIONAL HABILITATION PROGRAMS FOR
## THE DEVELOPMENTALLY DISABLED

### Vocational Habilitation

Vocational or pre-vocational services to out of school handicapped individuals are usually provided under the aegis of three service delivery systems:

1. adult activity centers
2. work activity centers
3. sheltered workshops

An adult activity facility, sometimes referred to as a day-treatment center is usually defined as a facility with a developmental program of structured training for the most severely involved clients. Adult activity programming would typically concentrate on eating skills, toilet training, communications, ambulation, and training in the most fundamental skills. It is generally assumed that individuals in adult activity centers or in day-training programs are so severely involved that vocational training is of a very low priority.

A work activity center is defined by the U.S. Department of Labor (Title 29, Chapter V, Part 525, May 17, 1974) in the following terms:

> Work activity center shall mean a workshop, or physically separated department of a workshop having an identifiable program, separate supervision and records, planned and designed exclusively to provide therapeutic activities for handicapped workers whose physical or mental impairment is so severe as to make their productive capacity inconsequential.

Work activity center clients are generally considered to be higher functioning than adult activity or day-treatment clients. Programming in work activity centers may also involve eating skills, toilet training, and the use of community transportation; however, programming in work activity centers is usually higher level and more social in nature and may involve weekly regimens of bowling, swimming, and craft work. Despite the assumed higher functioning level of work activity center clients, their productive capacity is still considered "inconsequential."

A legal definition of a sheltered workshop as stipulated by the U.S. Department of Labor (Title 29, Chapter V, Part 525, May 17, 1974) is:

> "Sheltered workshop" or "workshop" means a charitable organization or institution conducted not for profit but for the purpose of carrying out a recognized program of rehabilitation for handicapped workers, and/or providing such individuals rudimentary employment or other occupational rehabilitating activity of an educational or therapeutic nature.

Sheltered workshop employees are generally considered to be higher functioning individuals who are capable of doing complex work but require the structure of a sheltered environment in which to perform their activity. Sheltered workshops may be either long term (where the client's limitations are such that competitive employment is highly improbable) or transitional (where the client needs a sheltered supportive environment for a limited period of time). To qualify as a sheltered employee, the client must be able to produce at the level of one-half the productive capacity of a nonhandicapped worker and must be paid at a minimum of one-half of the prevailing federal wage in effect at the time of employment. Adult and work activity center clients, if they work at all, are usually paid on a piece rate because it is assumed that they are incapable of producing at a sheltered workshop level.

At face value, the concept of the adult, work, and sheltered workshop system is appealing. From a developmental standpoint, it makes sense to provide training that is based on the needs and on the functioning level of the individual client. However, there is evidence that the entire system of adult and work activity center and sheltered workshops may be flawed at two levels:

1.  Community adult and work activity centers and sheltered workshops may not be serving populations of an appropriate functioning level.
2.  The programming in these facilities may be questionable. A recent survey (Lynch and Gerber, 1977) of Michigan's adult, work activity, and sheltered workshops found a significant number of very high functioning individuals being provided services in adult and work activity centers.

As is evident from Table 1, a significant number of very high functioning clients are to be found in adult and work activity centers. Adult activity centers reported that the majority of their population (approximately 79%) function in the high-severe to low-mild range of retardation. Similarly, work activity centers reported that 85% of their

Table 1. Breakdown according to functioning level of population in adult activity, work activity, and sheltered workshop centers

| IQ | Adult activity center clients (%) | Work activity center clients (%) | Sheltered workshop center clients (%) |
|---|---|---|---|
| Over 80 | — | .6 | — |
| 66–80 | 7.2 | 15.2 | 55.9 |
| 50–65 | 22.3 | 40.2 | 23.1 |
| 35–49 | 49.0 | 31.0 | 16.7 |
| 20–34 | 12.2 | 11.4 | 2.9 |
| 0–19 | 9.3 | 1.6 | 1.4 |

population functions in the high-severe to low-mild range of retardation. It should be remembered that clients of this functioning level have been shown to be capable of learning and subsequently producing complex assembly tasks in real and experimental work situations. Assuming that clients served in Michigan's facilities are not unlike clients in other facilities throughout the United States, it is possible to suggest that there are many high functioning developmentally disabled adults now residing in community facilities that are designed to serve the needs of much lower functioning persons.

Survey data would also seem to indicate that programming received by the comparatively high functioning individuals in work and adult activity centers is also inadequate. As is evident in Table 2, fully 50% of the treatment day is spent in activities that could be construed to be infantilizing for mildly, moderately, and severely developmentally disabled adults.

Last, and most seriously, many adult and work activity centers erect admission barriers to acting-out and nontoilet trained individuals. While such admission barriers might be understandable in sheltered workshops, they are less understandable in work activity centers and inconceivable for adult activity centers.

As is evident in Table 1, sheltered workshops are serving comparatively few individuals below the mild range of retardation. These survey data would seem to be in agreement with those reported by Greenleigh and associates (1975) in their survey entitled, *The Role of the Sheltered Workshops in the Rehabilitation of the Severely Handicapped.* In light of the work capacity of the developmentally disabled client and in light of the work orientation of sheltered workshops, it is unfortunate that the developmentally disabled population is underrepresented. However, it has been suggested (Lynch, 1976) that sheltered workshops would be extremely hard pressed to provide work

Table 2.    Breakdown by percentage of program elements in vocational centers for the developmentally disabled

| Program element | Adult activity center (%) | Work activity center (%) | Sheltered workshop (%) |
|---|---|---|---|
| Recreation | 11.5 | 5.9 | — |
| Crafts | 31.9 | 49.3 | — |
| Contract work | — | 20.0 | 100 |
| Community survival skills | 48.0 | 20.3 | — |
| Free time | 8.6 | 4.5 | — |

skills training for the developmentally disabled because their orientation and experience is with much higher functioning individuals. Additionally, it has been suggested (Greenleigh, 1975) that many sheltered workshops have lost sight of their rehabilitation and training role in their attempts to generate contract revenue.

The concept of the adult and work activity centers carries with it a self-fulfilling prophecy that individuals enrolled in such programs are capable, at best, of only"inconsequential" work. As a result, many individuals who would be capable of high levels of satisfying and productive enterprise are given programming that is essentially infantilizing and that, perhaps, only contributes to the notion that developmentally disabled citizens are somehow vastly different from nonhandicapped individuals.

The belief that adult and work activity center clients are capable of only "inconsequential" production has also resulted in the development of a major barrier to the implementation of the 1973 Vocational Rehabilitation Act (P.L. 93-112). The 1973 Act has as its highest priority the delivery of rehabilitation and habilitation services to the severely handicapped. Under the provisions of the Act, funds may be made available for the evaluation, work adjustment, training, and placement of individuals capable of either competitive or sheltered employment. In the reinforcement system in which rehabilitation counselors work, the placement of a client in competitive employment is most highly prized while the placement of a client into sheltered employment is less highly regarded. However, under current regulations, the evaluation, training, and subsequent placement of a client into an adult or work activity center is generally regarded as a failure. As such, most rehabilitation counselors do not like to accept clients from adult and work activity centers since it is generally believed by rehabilitation counselors that the work capacity of these clients is "inconsequential." Additionally, clients residing in communities that do not have a licensed sheltered workshop are frequently denied evaluation and training services because rehabilitation counselors placing these clients into any setting other than competitive employment or a sheltered workshop will have their activity regarded as a failure.

## Vocational Education

The Vocational Education Amendments of 1968 (P.L. 90-567) were written with a view to emphasize the importance of making high quality vocational education services accessible to the severely handi-

capped. To that end, fully 10% of all federal funds spent under the Act
was to be used only for the cost of providing vocational education to
the handicapped. Despite the fact that it has been clearly
demonstrated that developmentally disabled workers can both be
trained and made productive, there is little evidence that this population, to any extent, is receiving services under the Act. In fact, unlike
Vocational Rehabilitation Services, vocational and technical education services do not require State Vocational Education Departments
to describe their treatment populations according to handicapping
conditions.

Because the field of vocational education is disinclined to serve
the developmentally disabled, the responsibility falls haphazardly on
the shoulders of special educators who, in all likelihood, may not have
a vocational orientation. As a result, preparation for productive and
responsible years after determination of school programming may be
nonexistent or of questionable value in that the disciplines that should
be training these clients may be unwilling or unable to do so. In light
of the productive capacity of the developmentally disabled and in light
of the potential contribution of vocational education funds and
technology to train this population, vocational-technical programs at
the state and community level should be compelled to recognize their
obligations to the developmentally disabled student.

It should be noted that many of the research studies cited earlier
and the majority of the work occurring at the Vocational Services
Component of the Institute for the Study of Mental Retardation and
Related Disabilities at the University of Michigan have been
conducted with the developmentally disabled clients who have never
received vocational education services and who seldom had had special education programming during school. Despite an almost total
lack of self concept as a worker and despite the absence of even the
most rudimentary concepts of job safety and job related behaviors,
these older clients have shown remarkable proficiency in task acquisition and subsequent production. Borrowing from the research on early
intervention and preschool programs, one can only speculate on how
these same clients might have performed if work concepts or specific
work skills were taught during the formative years.

At the present time, there is no conceptual model upon which to
base a vocational education curriculum for the developmentally disabled. A quality curriculum should be based on the known future needs
of the student and should attempt to provide the student with the skills
and abilities to succeed in that future environment. In light of the cur-

rent status of adult and work activity centers and sheltered workshops, it is clear that curriculum models could not, as a general rule, be based on performance criteria in those programs. New conceptual models need to be devised that are based on more realistic appraisals of the vocational capacity of the developmentally disabled.

As a minimum, school facilities for the developmentally disabled should feature a simulated workshop, with simulated work tasks, ranging from very simple color, form, size, and texture discriminations to very complex discriminations of the same order. Attending skills, high rates of error-free production, and appropriate work dress and general work behavior should be reinforced in a simulated workshop. Over a period of months and years, the students can be given an ever increasing simulated work day with increasing levels of responsibility and task complexity. In cooperation with local industry, "sheltered enclaves" would be developed wherein severely handicapped developmentally disabled clients could receive on-the-job training and subsequent placement after graduation from mandated school programs. Additionally, lower functioning developmentally disabled clients would receive on-the-job training and vocational and pre-vocational experiences in sheltered workshops, work activity centers, and adult activity centers. As was suggested earlier, of course, these facilities would be serving developmentally disabled clients in ways substantially unlike current practices.

Vocational education programming would also be concerned with the larger issue of teaching community survival skills which would enhance the sheltered or competitive vocational life of the client. Specifically, vocational education programming for the developmentally disabled would teach the use of community transportation. Furthermore, as many clients will be living in group homes, foster homes, and sheltered apartments, training should also be provided in the use of the washing machine and dryer, safety in the kitchen, basic shopping skills, and basic money management.

## CONCLUSION

In the past 5 to 10 years, the Department of Health, Education, and Welfare, state departments of education, and local communities have invested billions of dollars in the development and dissemination of early identification and intervention programs, and the building and staffing of specialized schools for the developmentally disabled child and youth. Children that, in an earlier day would have been institutionalized are now remaining in their local communities and are receiving programming that should result in the general increase in functional level. However, despite the national commitment to deinstitutionalization and the development of community services and facilities, there is one area of specific functioning that has not received programmatic attention, either in the school curriculum, or in the development of community facilities. This neglected area is the broad field of vocational education and vocational rehabilitation of the developmentally disabled. If the national commitment to the education of the developmentally disabled children is to be at all productive, it must now begin to deal with the inescapable conclusion that these children and youths will become adults.

## REFERENCES CITED

Bandura, A. 1969. Principles of Behavior Modification. Holt, Rinehart, and Winston, New York.

Bellamy, G. T., Inman, D. B., Swartz, Robert H. 1977. A review of habilitation techniques with the severely and profoundly retarded. In: N. Haring and D. Ricker (eds.), Teaching the Severely and Profoundly Handicapped, Volume 3. (In press).

Bellamy, G. T., Peterson, L., Close, D. 1975. Habilitation of the severely and profoundly retarded: Illustrations of competence. J. Ed. Train. Ment. Retard. 10:174–186.

Clarke, A. and Heremelin, F. 1955. Adult imbeciles: Their abilities and trainability. Lancet 2:337–339.

Crosson, J. E. 1966. The experimental analysis of vocational behavior in severely retarded males. Unpublished doctoral dissertation, University of Oregon.

Crosson, J. E. 1960. The functional analysis of behavior: A technology for special education practices. Ment. Retard. 7(4):15–19.

Flanders, J. P. 1968. A review of research on imitative behavior, Psychol. Bull., Vol. 69(5):316–337.

Gold, M. W. 1974. Redundant cue removal in skill training for the retarded. Ed. Train. of the Ment. Retard. 9(1):5–8.

Gold, M. W. 1973. Research on the vocational habilitation of the retarded: The present and the future. In N. Ellis (ed.), International Review of Research in Mental Retardation, Vol. 6 Academic Press, New York.

Gold, M. W. 1972. Stimulus factors in skill training of the retarded on a complex assembly task: Acquisition, transfer, and retention. Am. J. Ment. Defic. 76:517–526.

Gold, M. W. and Barclay, C. R. 1975. The effects of verbal labels on the acquisition and retention of complex assembly tasks. Train. Sch. Bull. 70:39–43.

Greenleigh Associates, 1975. The role of the sheltered workshop in the rehabilitation of the severely handicapped. Executive Summary, Vol. 1., Washington, D.C.

Loos, F. and Tizard, J. 1955. The employment of adult imbeciles in a hospital workshop. Am. J. Ment. Defic. 59:395–403.

Lynch, K. P. 1976. Vocational programming for the developmentally disabled. Presented at the American Association on Mental Deficiency Conference in Chicago.

Lynch, K. P. and Gerber, P. 1977. A survey of adult services to the developmentally disabled in Michigan. University of Michigan, Ann Arbor. (In press).

Lynch, K. P. and Malian, I. M. 1977. Comparative effectiveness of a reinforced video modeling procedure in teaching a complex assembly task to a population of severely handicapped individuals. University of Michigan, Ann Arbor. (In press).

The role of the sheltered workshops in the rehabilitation of the severely handicapped. Vol. 1. Greenleigh Associates, 1975, Washington, D.C.

Wolfensberger, W. 1967. Vocational preparation and occupation. In: A. Baumeister (ed.), Mental Retardation. Alden Atherton, Chicago.

*Wyatt v. Aderholt*, 334 F. Supp. 1341 (N.D. Alabama, 1971), 325 F. Supp. 781 (N.D. Alabama, 1971).

# chapter eleven

# SEX EDUCATION

Vivien Dee, R.N., M.N.

The current emphasis on the sexual and human rights of the developmentally disabled and the desire for their integration into the community has brought new challenges to health care professionals who work with them.

Many of the problems facing developmentally disabled adolescents are not different from those of the normal adolescent, but because of their handicaps and restricted environment, opportunities for social interaction and development are limited. Their chances to observe, develop, and practice social skills are often nonexistent. The lack of peer reference groups and the inability to validate the accuracy of what limited sex information may be available through older adolescents in the community only adds to the developmentally disabled adolescents' lack of acceptable social conduct.

In the American sociocultural system sex education is the responsibility of parents who are the primary source of information for their children; however, many parents tend to procrastinate and if possible avoid providing any information to their children. Parents often do not prepare themselves to meet all the sexual and social educational needs of their developmentally disabled adolescents. Many parents are anxious, uncomfortable, and embarrassed, and therefore, avoid the discussion of sexual issues. This type of guidance is then left for others to do.

Nurses, along with other health professionals and educators, must prepare themselves with the information and the training necessary to teach effectively and to initiate explanations at a level best understood by the developmentally disabled. They must have the ability to examine their own attitudes about sexuality as well as their attitudes toward the developmentally disabled adolescents in day to day living experiences.

Although the role of the nurse as a sex educator and counselor has not been fully explored or developed, it is recommended that the nurse familiarize herself with the intrafamily relationships and attitudes about sex, anticipate and emphasize the needs of the developmentally disabled adolescent for the parents at various stages of his development, suggest appropriate times for providing sex information, recommend approaches for teaching or counselling, and educate or re-educate parents, other professionals, and the community for greater acceptance of the sexual humanism of the developmentally disabled.

Nurses working at Development Centers, Residential Treatment Facilities, and community programs such as school and outpatient clinics, have the responsibility for dispelling misconceptions about, on the one hand, the developmentally disabled individual's lack of sexual needs, and on the other, his supposed sexual agressiveness.

Although sex education becomes imperative during the adolescent years primarily because of the onset of pubertal changes and its emerging sexuality, sex education must begin from the individual's birth and it is a life-long process.

Since much sexual knowledge is imparted to the developmentally disabled adolescent through nonverbal communication, and behavior and attitudes of parents toward each other, the nurse must assist the parents in exploring their own personal values and beliefs regarding sexuality.

It is essential to involve parents in the sex education of their adolescents as:

1.  an observer of their adolescent's behaviors
2.  a teacher in the home
3.  a provider for new social experiences
4.  a model for socially appropriate behaviors

The goal of any sex education program should be to help developmentally disabled adolescents and their parents to deal with questions, dilemmas, and problems related to sexuality.

## SEXUALITY OF THE DEVELOPMENTALLY DISABLED

### Misconceptions and Fears

In the past, the general societal attitude toward the developmentally disabled has not been favorable, or accepting. Individuals who differed from others in some aspect like beauty or intellect were viewed as deviants. Deviant individuals were therefore consciously perceived or labeled as subhumans, animal-like, or "vegetables." Because of the subhuman label, these individuals were stripped of their rights and privileges as human beings.

A deviant individual was seen as a public menace because of his alleged contribution to genetic decline; he was to be punished or ostracized in order to protect the society. Or a deviant individual was viewed as an object of pity, likely to be held blameless for his condition, unaccountable for his behavior, and exempted from normal social responsibilities.

Deviancies were believed to be associated with retardation and responsible for conditions and illnesses such as alcoholism, physical impediments, poverty, prostitution, epilepsy, crime, illegitimacy, vagrancy, and mental illness. Society's efforts to handle deviancy concentrated on institutionalizing these individuals, thereby removing them from interaction with their families and the community. Problems of sexual and social behavior were largely ignored, except pregnancy, in which case an abortion or sterilization was performed.

Such perceptions and attitudes were the basis for some of the following misconceptions and fears about the developmentally disabled, who were viewed as objects of deviance because of their differentness in biological, intellectual, social, and physical development:

1. the developmentally disabled should not marry
2. the developmentally disabled have no sexual feelings and are incapable of heterosexual relationships
3. the developmentally disabled are sexually aggressive and dangerous
4. the developmentally disabled would be exploited by immoral men in the community

Although the sexual behavior of the developmentally disabled has been of great concern to many, comparatively little research is available to guide professionals and parents in understanding the sexuality of the developmentally disabled. A review of literature reveals the following information and facts about the sexuality of the developmentally disabled.

**Some Facts**

1. The developmentally disabled have sexual drives and interest in the opposite sex; however, the heterosexual interest is lower as the level of intellectual functioning decreases.
2. Sexual offenses are usually of a harmless character, such as public masturbation and indecent exposure. There seems to be a correlation between sexual offenses and general inadequacy.

3.  Psychosexual maturation occurs at a later chronological age as compared to persons of normal intelligence.

4.  Sex role recognition is greater for the older adolescent who comes closer to his normal peer in level of overall functioning than the younger or more severely developmentally disabled adolescent.

5.  The average age at which the developmentally disabled reach physiological maturation is 13.3 years, essentially the same as normal pubescence.

6.  Delayed pubescence is more frequent when the disability is prenatal or genetic in origin.

7.  Difficulties in motor coordination, family restrictions or activities, and lack of social exposure contribute to the lag in identification with sex roles.

8.  The behavior of the moderately and the more severely developmentally disabled adolescents are basically exploratory and characteristic of younger children.

9.  Mildly developmentally disabled adolescents express a desire to date, seek out companionship, and ask questions about sex.

10. Many developmentally disabled individuals are unable to express feelings, possibly because they do not see themselves as recipients of symbolic or concrete affection.

11. Females receive sex education more often than males, primarily because of the onset of menarche.

12. The greater the degree of mental deficiency, the slower the development of secondary sex characteristics.

13. The developmentally disabled individuals have difficulty foreseeing the consequences of their acts.

14. The sexual expression and behavior of the severely developmentally disabled can be at the level of auto-eroticism.

15. Genital manipulation and masturbation are often fostered by boredom, lack of activities, and a failure to understand what is acceptable social conduct.

16. The higher the intellectual functioning of the developmentally disabled, the greater is his ability to sustain a reasonably successful marriage with no children or at most with one child.

17. The developmentally disabled adolescent in institutions demonstrate less knowledge on sociosexual topics as compared to developmentally disabled adolescents living at home.

18. The progeny of mothers with IQs below 67 have a 14-fold increase in the probability of having a child with an IQ below 67 as compared to those with a mother whose IQ is at or above 100.

## RIGHTS OF THE DEVELOPMENTALLY DISABLED

In recent years, national interest in all aspects of work on behalf of the developmentally disabled has contributed to the social redefinition of deviancy and the redetermination of the role and status of the handicapped. This process has stimulated new directions in social policy and greater understanding and acceptance of the developmentally disabled. As society's perceptions of deviancy changed, increased recognition and pursuance of the rights of the developmentally disabled ensued. These include:

1. right to treatment and habilitation services
2. right to dignity, privacy, and humane care
3. right to participate in an appropriate program of publicly supported education, regardless of degree of handicap
4. right to prompt medical care and treatment
5. right to religious freedom and practice
6. right to social interaction and participation in community activities
7. right to physical exercise and recreational opportunities
8. right to be free from harm, including unnecessary physical restraint, or isolation, excessive medication, abuse, or neglect
9. right to be free from hazardous procedures[1]

Although major emphasis on the procurement of rights for the developmentally disabled has been on humane care and treatment, little has been heard about the personal rights of these individuals; the right to marry, the right to sexual freedom outside marriage, the right to bear children, the right to raise children and the right to family life. Nurses working in the area of sexual counseling and sex education must be prepared to discuss the ethical issues concerning these rights and their implications.

The growing acceptance of the normalization principle, that each individual should be integrated into society on a personal level through normal avenues of interaction, has brought on a greater need for preparing the developmentally disabled individuals for this process, primarily because they are less well equipped to handle the complexities of the demands made by the society.

Sex education and sexual counseling is one means of preparing these individuals toward social integration.

---

[1] Lanterman Developmental Disabilities Services ACT, Assembly Bill 3800, State of California.

The objectives of sex education are to:

1.  promote positive self image
2.  promote social adjustment and acceptable behaviors
3.  promote self-care behaviors
4.  provide accurate information

The following concepts must guide the nurse in the sex education of every developmentally disabled individual:

1.  the developmentally disabled can and do learn
2.  the developmentally disabled's learning ability varies from person to person
3.  the developmentally disabled has the right to reach the highest level of development sexually and socially
4.  sexual training must be done within the total framework of training for life
5.  sex education includes the issues of reproduction, anatomical differences between male and female, but also all areas of human sexuality, including attitudes, feelings, and relationships

## ASSESSMENT

The development of a program of sex education or sexual counseling must be based on the assessed needs of the developmentally disabled adolescent. His sexual knowledge, attitudes, level of intellectual functioning, and his biopsychosexual maturation must be considered in order to guide him toward appropriate sexual expression and social expectation.

Assessment involves not only clarifying and identifying present difficulties but also past trends and desired future behavior in terms of his social adjustment. It involves an analysis of many aspects of the developmentally disabled adolescents' life to determine the nature of the problem, the reasons for it, and the prospects for dealing with it.

Assessment should be a continuous process and must be based on a developmental continuum framework.

### Purposes

The purposes of assessment are to:

1.  determine the characteristics of the learner
2.  determine the kind of approach to use in teaching

3. determine the learner's readiness for learning
4. determine the depth of content materials
5. determine priorities for teaching or counseling

## Method

Assessing the needs of the developmentally disabled adolescent can be accomplished in a variety of ways, such as observation, verbal communication, and the use of a variety of assessment tools.

Direct observation of the adolescent's behavior can be done in structured situations (e.g., classrooms, sheltered workshops) or in unstructured situations (e.g., clinic waiting rooms, homes). Observing his interactions with his peers, parents, and other adults can provide the following information: 1) his own behavioral repertoire, 2) the extent of his limitations resulting from physical disability, and 3) his parents' reaction to his behaviors, whether appropriate or inappropriate.

Verbal communication with the adolescent may be accomplished by utilizing either an unstructured technique of allowing the adolescent to report on his own thoughts and feelings, or through a more structured technique of questions and answers.

Visual aids such as dolls and picture booklets may be used to elicit information from adolescents who are less able to provide subjective reporting or respond to a question and answer format.

Frequently, with the more developmentally disabled adolescent, parents are seen before the adolescent. This process is helpful because it allows parents to share ways of eliciting information from the adolescents as well as to provide pertinent information regarding the social adjustment of their children.

This process is also helpful because it communicates to parents what information will be obtained or given to their child. It alleviates parental anxieties that discussion of sexual matters may "stimulate" or preoccupy the adolescent's mind with sex. It allows the parents to become aware of the nature and extent of their adolescent's learning needs, and provides an opportunity for parents to discuss:

1. their own attitudes regarding sex education
2. their own expectations regarding their adolescent's independent living, vocational choice, marriage, etc.
3. how they deal with sexual issues and social behaviors of their child
4. their own feelings, values and beliefs and how these are communicated to the adolescent

## Individual Assessment

Although the developmentally disabled are generally grouped into three categories—mild, moderate and severely developmentally disabled, based on their level of intelligence—many of them differ in their capacity to communicate, in their ability to accept responsibility, in their home environment, and in the availability of support systems. Failure to recognize their individual unique strengths and weaknesses often limits their potential for growth and development. The more each individual's specific abilities and disabilities are recognized, the more tailored will be the programs to meet his particular pattern of abilities and disabilities. With this framework in mind, it becomes essential that an individual assessment be done prior to planning a program of training or counseling for the developmentally disabled.

The factors listed below include some of the suggested areas for assessment but are not intended to be all inclusive:

1) Level of intellectual functioning:
   a) level of ability to follow instructions?
   b) level of reading ability and comprehension?
   c) level of ability to retain information?
   d) span of attention?
2) Physical disabilities and limitations:
   a) Are senses intact or defective, e.g., vision, hearing?
   b) What is his mode of communication, through speech or gestures?
   c) What is the level of gross and fine motor coordination?
   d) Are limitations imposed by physical disability?
3) Stage of biopsychosexual maturation:
   a) stage of pubertal development? Has menses started? secondary sex development?
   b) Does he express curiosity in the opposite sex?
   c) Does he have a special friend, same sex or opposite sex?
   d) Does the awareness of anatomical differences arouse sexual feelings?
   e) Is he able to differentiate sexual advances from normal friendly encounters?
4) Awareness of physical differences and sex roles:
   a) What sex role does he identify with, same sex or opposite sex?
   b) What does he know about the anatomical differences of the sexes?

    c)  Does he have opportunity to see immature or mature male or female genitalia?

5)  Mode of sexual expression:
    a)  How does he express his feeling when he is sad, angry, happy?
    b)  How does he display affection?
    c)  Is his show of affection directed toward family members, familiar adults or strangers?
    d)  Are sexual interest and expression directed toward same sex, opposite sex, or self, e.g., masturbation?

6)  Types of social experiences:
    a)  Who are his friends? Same or opposite sex?
    b)  With whom does he spend most of his time, or does he spend it alone?
    c)  What kind of social activities does he engage in? Bowling, dancing?
    d)  With mixed groups or same sex groups?
    e)  Are activities supervised or unsupervised?
    f)  What is his living condition or situation like? At home? In a foster home, or residential facility?
    g)  Are his social behaviors adaptive to age or societal norms?

**Establishing Priorities**

At the completion of the assessment process, identified problems must be ranked or ordered according to their magnitude, importance, and consequences to the developmentally disabled adolescent. Some needs require resources such as social groups and recreational facilities for the adolescent to observe, develop, and practice social skills. Some needs require other clinical expertise involving medical procedures and examinations, such as issues related to contraception, pregnancy, and sexual development. Some needs require individual attention and training since progress for the developmentally disabled is slow and some skills may be so complex that they need to be subdivided. Some needs can be met by anyone on the scene, for instance, parents in the home situation or teachers in the school settings. Finding learning situations where the adolescent can experience maximal success will help him to develop self-esteem. Some needs will resolve themselves when proper actions are taken, for instance, in situations where genital manipulation or masturbation becomes a problem, other possible causes should be investigated. Clothing should be considered, e.g., tight fitting pants should be replaced with looser pants; other conditions, such as infection in the genital or pubic area or uncleanliness, could be a cause of irritation and itching, in which case medical attention should be sought. Some needs and behaviors require specific guidelines and instructions so that detrimental consequences for these acts will be avoided.

## APPROACHES FOR TEACHING

The nurse as sex educator or counselor must be flexible in utilizing multiple approaches in a variety of learning situations. For the purpose of clarification the types of approaches are described separately, although in practice they are not mutually exclusive. The approaches are useful both for individuals and group teaching or counseling.

### Groups versus Individual

Group teaching is usually recommended for the mild to moderately developmentally disabled adolescent because it allows for individual members to share ideas in a reciprocal relationship and enhances the development of comradeship, peer support, and socialization. Interest level and group participation are often maintained when adolescents are selected for a group according to similar intellectual capabilities and equivalent psychosexual maturation.

For the mild to moderately developmentally disabled adolescent, the use of visual aids can provide a comfortable entry into the discussion of sexuality. The discussion of sex roles, dating behaviors, friendship, selection of mate, feelings, and opinions can be shared in a group situation. Similar approaches are used for the more moderately developmentally disabled, but content is kept on the concrete level rather than on an abstract level and the group format may be more structured including formal instruction.

Group teaching, however, is not recommended for the severely developmentally disabled since many of the necessary social skills and self-care skills are too complex and need to be broken down into small sequential steps. Instruction is therefore best provided on a one-to-one basis. Individual teaching and counseling may be applicable for all levels of developmentally disabled individuals who need individual attention for a specific kind of difficulty.

### Types of Approaches

*Natural Approach* This approach utilizes naturally occurring events in the individual's life experiences. This type of teaching is done informally and draws upon real life situations as a reference for learning for all levels of developmentally disabled individuals.

Although the use of picture booklets may be used initially for the purpose of directing attention, eliciting information, and teaching concepts to the moderate to severely developmentally disabled adolescent, eventually emphasis must be placed on finding learning situations as closely related to real life situations as possible. For instance, in teaching identification and recognition of body parts, continued suggestions must be made to him to identify his own body parts while bathing, toileting, dressing, and undressing. This approach allows for frequent practice sessions, reduces the need for an additional structured habilitative program in the course of the day, and provides a means of associating learned concepts to real life activities.

Since many of the mildly developmentally disabled adolescents are able to identify and recognize their body parts by using colloquial terms, teaching efforts are directed toward replacing the colloquial terms with the use of appropriate terminology, e.g., breast for "boobs" and penis for "ding-a-ling."

Similar approaches are used when acquainting the mild to moderately developmentally disabled adolescent females with their own genitalia, whether in preparation for the insertion of tampons during menstrual periods or in preparation for pelvic exams. The use of a mirror to view the genitalia while squatting allows for viewing of the three orifices, vagina, urethra, and anus, and an explanation of the function of each. It is unrealistic to expect the severely developmentally disabled adolescent female to perform this type of learning experience since it is unlikely that she will develop menstrual self care capability.

On the subject of the reproductive process, showing how familiar animals such as dogs and cats copulate can provide a natural way of absorbing ideas of mating for the moderately developmentally disabled adolescent. Differences in social behaviors and responsibility level between animals and humans must be presented, however, so that the student understands that humans copulate in private and have the responsibility of caring for their young.

Feelings of security, approval, self-esteem, and belonging cannot be taught solely in a structured classroom setting. Parents and teachers can help the mild to moderately developmentally disabled adolescent develop a positive concept of self by assigning tasks which he can perform successfully. Social activities such as family gatherings and recreational programs where he can practice his social skills and participate with relative success will enhance feelings of achievement and help him to achieve a sense of belonging and acceptance. Grooming and dressing in teenage fashion will help to promote his self-image and general well-being.

Since physical stimulation and social contacts are often minimal and restricted for the severely developmentally disabled, it is important for the nurse to be cognizant of the basic needs of the adolescent who is severely developmentally disabled, including the needs for comfort, warmth, and attention. The severely developmentally disabled adolescent is taught a greater appreciation and awareness of his body as a source for and a receiver of pleasurable experiences through touching, holding, changing diapers, talking, etc, even though little or no response may be observed initially by the nurse. Input that is pleasurable will eventually elicit behavior on the part of the adolescent.

*Preventive Approach*     This approach emphasizes the prevention of problems through the identification of peak periods in the life of the developing individual and the provision of guidance prior to the arrival of these peak periods. Guidance, either through instruction or counseling, is provided for the adolescent in efforts to assist him through various stages of his development with the least amount of emotional upheaval and trauma. This type of anticipatory guidance can be provided for all levels of developmentally disabled individuals.

The onset of menses is often a frightening experience for some of the mild to moderately developmentally disabled adolescent girls. The preventive approach or anticipatory guidance is recommended for girls approaching menarche. Preliminary instructions on identifying blood on sheets or night clothes can alleviate some of the fears associated with punishment or "sickness." Items used for menstrual care such as sanitary napkins, sanitary belts, or tampons can be introduced at this time to provide a beginning association for later use. Menstruation should be explained as a natural process for girls "growing up."

Similar anticipatory guidance should be provided for boys regarding nocturnal emissions, or "wet dreams." Explanations must be made that such biological discharges are healthy and a natural process for boys "growing up."

Since many of the more developmentally disabled adolescents have difficulty in retaining information or with the transference of learning, this type of anticipatory guidance is usually provided after the appearance of secondary sex characteristics, e.g., breast buds, pubic hair, etc.

Although it is helpful to prepare the moderate to severely developmentally disabled adolescent in advance for the changes which will occur, it is unrealistic to expect them to fully understand the reasons for such preparation.

Teaching social behaviors can be done in an informal way early in the adolescent's developing years. Behaviors such as common courtesy in greeting, learning to take turns, respecting privacy of self and others, for example, dressing or undressing in private quarters, or using the bathroom with the door closed, will assist the adolescent in achieving greater social acceptability. These social behaviors can be modeled in the home setting by parents or substitute parents.

For the maturing mildly developmentally disabled adolescent females, who have greater access to social exposure and heterosexual relationships, counseling and guidance should be provided in the area of contraceptive measures. The visits to the physician must be arranged to provide a beginning acquaintance with medical check ups and pelvic exams. Preparation for pelvic exam is provided so as not to alarm the adolescent. Similar approaches may be taken for moderately developmentally disabled females even though their social contacts may be limited and the start of interest in the opposite sex delayed.

***Social Learning Approach***   The social learning approach utilizes the principles of behavior modification in teaching all levels of developmentally disabled individuals self-care and social skills.

For all developmentally disabled adolescents, skills that are complex must be broken down into small sequential steps. For instance, in teaching menstrual self-care, the skills can be divided into five different components: 1) recognition of blood, 2) application of sanitary pad, 3) disposal of sanitary pad, 4) grooming and hygiene, and 5) monthly calendar.

Depending on the intellectual level of the developmentally disabled adolescent, each component may have to be broken down further into small sequential steps for the moderately developmentally disabled adolescent as in the application of the sanitary pad:

1. wash hands
2. sit down
3. draw belt up over the knees with tab fasteners centered between the legs
4. remove pad from box
5. place pad on lap with absorbant side facing up

6. gauze from back end is lifted up
7. twist the end of the tab
8. pick up tab fastener
9. push twisted tab through the large hole from below the fastener in an upward direction
10. pull the tab up against the prongs to secure it
11. repeat step 6–10 to secure the other end of the pad to the tab fastener[2]

Upon the completion of each step, it is immediately reinforced by a reward such as praise or a hug, in order to increase the probability of the behavior being repeated. As each step is learned the reward may be less frequently given. The selection of a reward must be personally reinforcing to the individual.

Unacceptable social behaviors such as genital exposure, masturbation, undressing, or lifting skirts up in public places should be discouraged. Simply to ignore masturbating in public places may not be the correct method for discouraging this behavior for a number of reasons: 1) masturbation is a behavior that is pleasurable and intrinsically rewarding and is not necessarily maintained by extrinsic rewards, 2) the adolescent may not be aware of the social consequences and legal implication of this behavior, and 3) the adolescent may not be aware that there are other places where he can masturbate acceptably and safely.

The recommended approach is to show disapproval verbally with an emphatic, "No, No," or "This is not the place to masturbate." It is not necessary to apply punitive measures such as slapping his fingers or shaming him; however, depending on the intellectual level of the developmentally disabled adolescent, he may have to be instructed repeatedly or even be shown private places—the bedroom, bathroom, or any other private quarters where he can masturbate safely. In addition, it is necessary to evaluate the amount of time he spends masturbating. Excessive periods of masturbation may suggest boredom, lack of activities, or loneliness. He must also learn to delay or postpone sexual gratification. He should be given social reinforcement when he refrains from masturbating in public places.

Similar approaches can be applied to discouraging genital exposure, undressing, or lifting skirts in public. The developmentally

---

[2] Adapted from Pattulo, A. 1969. Puberty in the Girl who is Retarded. National Association for Retarded Children, Arlington, Texas.

disabled adolescent must receive information on what behaviors will bring about attention in a positive way, in contrast to those behaviors which although calling attention to the adolescent, have detrimental consequences.

For the mild to moderately developmentally disabled adolescent, role playing as in creating or recreating a dating situation can provide practice sessions for developing social skills in the area of dating. Other social behaviors such as walking, sitting, and standing can be best accomplished through the use of observational learning as in modeling and imitation for developing poise.

## Parental Involvement

Any successful program requires a coordinated effort on the part of many individuals. The nurse as coordinator is responsible for assisting parents and teachers in developing knowledge of these approaches and how they are utilized. Nurses need to be aware that inherent in all these approaches are attitudes, feelings, and thoughts so often conveyed to the adolescent either intentionally or unintentionally through facial expressions, gestures, vocal tones and inflections. Counseling sessions with parents should have the following objectives:

1.  to help parents work through their own feelings and fears about the sexuality of the developmentally disabled
2.  to help parents sort out problem areas and get to the source of their concerns without becoming unduly alarmed
3.  to encourage parents to make a practice of evaluating situations where "sexual behavior" may occur
4.  to encourage parents to take initiative in discussing general issues of sexuality with their adolescents
5.  to help parents with a variety of approaches for teaching
6.  to help parents find learning situations
7.  to help parents set realistic goals for their developmentally disabled adolescents

## Curriculum

The curriculum, shown on Table 1, is divided into the following four major areas:

1.  awareness of self-emphasizing the individual in reference to his environment and to other persons around him
2.  physical changes and understanding of self-emphasizing the bodily

Table 1.   A curriculum guide for sex education of developmentally disabled adolescents[a]

| I. Awareness of self | II. Physical changes and understanding of self | III. Peer relationships | IV. Responsibility to society |
|---|---|---|---|
| A. Environment<br>1. Response of parent or substitute parent<br>2. Physical comfort from holding, bathing, feeling, changing<br>3. Emotional comfort: warm response from parent in spite of the lack of response<br>4. Stimulation from playing, movement, vocalization, etc.<br>5. Spatial awareness<br>B. Recognition of body parts, e.g., hand, ears, tummy, nose, etc.<br>1. Responds to naming of body parts through gesture or movement<br>2. Beginning awareness of relationship between use of article and body parts, e.g., soap, washcloth. | A. Sexual differences (physical-external)<br>1. Boys, e.g. genitals, penis, scrotum<br>2. Girls, e.g. breasts, vulva, vagina, etc.<br>B. Identification with like-sex and understanding of opposite sex:<br>1. Activities<br>2. Dress<br>3. Interpersonal relationships with one parent or substitute parent of like sex.<br>4. Masculine or feminine work responsibilities in home.<br>5. School expectation<br>C. Social role of child<br>1. In the family<br>a. family composition. | A. Development of self-respect<br>1. Success in achievement<br>2. Attention to appearance<br>3. Privacy-information<br>4. Self control<br>5. Acceptance of responsibility<br>6. Poise<br>B. Respect for others<br>1. Property rights<br>2. Privacy<br>3. Opinions<br>4. Feelings<br>C. Peer expectations<br>1. Influence of individuals<br>2. Influence of groups<br>3. Behavior of friendships<br>D. Responsibility to group<br>1. Using group for support | A. Single life<br>1. Independent living<br>2. Social relations<br>B. Preparation for marriage<br>C. Selection of a mate<br>D. Financial obligations of marriage<br>E. Husband–wife relations<br>F. Contraception<br>G. Responsibility for care of a household<br>H. Child care |

b. purposes of family group
c. parent-child relationship
d. sibling relationship

2. Beyond family
   a. extended family
   b. peers
   c. other adults
   d. organized activities

D. Awareness of individual differences
   1. Physical
      a. Height
      b. Weight
      c. Size
      d. Appearance
   2. Behavioral
      a. Personality characteristics
   3. Intellectual limitations and abilities
   4. Family likeness
      a. In growth and development
      b. In appearance

2. Using group as a challenge
3. Need of success in group
4. Concern for good of group

E. Prelude to group relations
   1. Courtesy
   2. Thoughtfulness
   3. Values of rights of individuals
   4. Values of group membership
   5. Standards of behavior
   6. Self discipline

F. Identification with same and opposite sex
   1. Sex roles

G. Acceptance of changing role in relation to others
   1. The family as a societal unit.
      a) family problems
      b) Sibling relationships
      c) Rights of individuals of family

C. Identification of body processes, e.g., eating, sleeping, elimination
   1. Awareness of "getting ready to eat," "going to the bathroom," habit training.
   2. Awareness of relationship between use of equipment or facility associated with body process, e.g., elimination—potty, bed pan, bathroom.

D. Toilet training
   1. Beginning use of appropriate terminology
   2. Establishing schedule.
   3. Use of appropriate facility (e.g., toilet-ing-bathroom)
   4. Management of clothing.

*Continued*

Table 1—*Continued*

| I. Awareness of self | II. Physical changes and understanding of self | III. Peer relationships | IV. Responsibility to society |
|---|---|---|---|
| E. Identification of body parts: e.g., head, abdomen, nose, mouth, penis, buttocks, etc.<br>1. Appropriate use of name of body parts | E. Preparation for changes in self<br>1. Origin of life<br>2. Understanding pubertal changes<br>  a. Boys: | d) Responsibilities of individuals<br>H. Acceptance of role as an employee<br>1. Subordinate role | |
| F. Independent care of body needs<br>1. Hygienic needs, e.g., wiping nose, brushing teeth, washing face, etc.<br>2. Eating—feeding<br>3. Dressing |     1) Broadening of shoulders<br>    2) Growth of hair on face, pubic area, arm pits<br>    3) Skin<br>    4) Later growth spurts |   a) Boy with female boss<br>  b) Boy with male boss<br>  c) Girl with male boss<br>  d) Girl with female boss | |
| G. Attitudes toward body<br>1. Beginning participation in activities within capacity. |     5) Muscular development<br>    6) Change in voice | I. Social relationships<br>1. Heterosexual<br>  a) Preparation for dating | |
| H. Verbalization of feelings in response to gross stimulation, e.g., "itch", pain, scratchy, etc. |     7) Development of reproductive system |   b) Selection of companion<br>  c) Arranging for date | |
| I. Awareness of self in relation to others<br>1. As a family member<br>2. As a group member | |   d) Accepting a date<br>  e) Dating behavior e.g., courtesy, petting, etc. | |

J. Awareness of emotional self and basic needs for
  1. Security
  2. Social approval
  3. Belonging and acceptance
  4. Self-esteem
  5. Achievement
  6. Affection
  7. Independence

K. Awareness of self as a person capable of influencing others

F. Acceptance of change
  1. Observes changes in others
  2. Compares self with others
  3. Has ego strength to accept his status.

G. Changes in relationships and social expectation
  1. Change role
  2. Increase responsibility.

H. Emotional response to like sex and opposite sex

I. Conception
  1. Reproductive purposes
  2. Review of male and female reproductive organs
  3. Act of intercourse
  4. Contraception
  5. Social implications

J. Pregnancy
  1. Selection of a doctor
  2. Following doctor's directions

J. Premarital intercourse
  1. Abstinence
  2. Double standard

a Taken from *A Resource Guide in Sex Education For The Mentally Retarded*. Reprinted by permission of: Unit of Progress of the Handicapped in cooperation with the association for the Advancement of Health Education, an Association of the American Alliance for Health, Physical Education and Recreation and the Sex Information and Education Council of the United States.

changes which occur during puberty, the emotional adjustment and interpersonal relationships

3. peer relationships—emphasizing the individual's responsibility as a member of groups and the influence of peers

4. responsibility to society—emphasizing the social and biological implications of marriage

The curriculum is intended as a guide for sex education. It is presented as a continuum beginning with concepts related to self followed by concepts related to self and others. Under each major area are concepts with increasing difficulty as well as concepts that overlap into other major areas.

Concepts under each major area are taught interchangably depending on the immediate needs of the individual. For instance, a developmentally disabled female who is sexually active may first need to be counseled on the use of contraceptive measures and immediately after this is accomplished other areas including feelings of approval, self-esteem, peer relationships, and social behaviors are considered.

Teaching must begin with specific and simple concepts, moving on to more complex concepts as the individual is able to comprehend them. For instance, in discussing sex roles, discussion may begin with traditional roles, including specific tasks and duties identified as feminine or masculine. When the individual is able to comprehend and conceptualize these traditional roles, discussion may proceed to more current changes in society and their effects on feminine and male roles.

Another example may be taken when explaining the menses. Teaching begins with simple concept of health and self-care, as in the application of sanitary pads described earlier. As the student becomes capable of understanding more, the biological aspects of the menses can be discussed, leading on to discussing peer relationships as in womanhood and manhood, heterosexual relationships, and eventually, the social and biological implications of marriage or independent single living.

As a guideline, emphasis is placed on teaching the severely developmentally disabled adolescent areas related to self and basic self-care and social behavior. For the moderately and mildly developmentally disabled adolescent, teaching may include the following areas: 1) awareness of self, 2) physical changes and understanding of self, and 3) peer relationships.

For the mildly developmentally disabled adolescent, topics

related to marriage and child care are presented during late adolescence. Teaching efforts are directed toward maximizing each individual's potential for productive and independent living. It is realistic, however, to assume that many will not be able to lead fully independent lives with responsibility for care of a household. Each individual's level of intellectual and physical abilities and potential should be taken into consideration when planning a program of sex education.

## Case Illustration

*Case 1*    Lisa, age 17, was a moderately developmentally disabled adolescent female. She was the oldest of three children. Her two younger siblings consisted of a half brother and a half sister. The etiology of her developmental disability was not known.

Lisa was attending a school for the trainable mentally retarded at the time of her referral to the clinic. She was referred by her teachers for help because of her frequent hand touching behaviors toward her classmates. She was also yelling "dirty" words and propositioning her peers with "Let's go to bed." These activities were not only disruptive in the classroom, but also alarming to the teachers.

Mrs. C., Lisa's mother, was seen at the clinic and essentially provided the same information and validated the teacher's concern. She was interviewed first and provided information regarding Lisa's learning abilities, their home situation, and her own fears for Lisa. She requested that Lisa be sterilized.

Upon further interviewing, Mrs. C. provided the following information. She was divorced from her first husband shortly after the confirmation of Lisa's diagnosis. She later remarried someone belonging to the same church. Mrs. C. was a devout Catholic and continued to attend church with her family. During the 5 months prior to the referral, church attendance had become unbearable primarily because of Lisa's embarrassing social behaviors. In addition, other family problems emerged. Mike, Lisa's 14-year-old half brother, refused to attend classes. Mr. C. had been pressuring Mrs. C. to "get rid of" Lisa.

Out of sheer desperation and the lack of alternative approaches and knowledge, Mrs. C. was asking for sterilization as a means of controlling Lisa's social behavior and sexual desires.

Lisa was seen next. She was dressed a few years younger than her stated age of 17. She was able to respond to her name and a few questions regarding her schooling and home life. She was able to state simply and briefly her reason for coming to the clinic. According to her, she was to learn how to behave in class.

In order to develop a program for modifying Lisa's touching behavior, it was necessary to determine the frequency of these occurrences. An observation period was imperative. It was arranged with the classroom teacher that she observe and record the number of times Lisa actually touched one of her fellow classmates. This recording showed an average of one per minute. A program of intervention was established utilizing the social learning approach in the classroom.

Upon conferring with both Mrs. C. and the classroom teacher, it was decided that social praise was personally reinforcing for Lisa. Therefore, Lisa was instructed that if she were to refrain from touching any of her fellow classmates for a designated period of time, she would be commended by her teacher with "Lisa, that's ladylike." Small increments of time period were established for reinforcement purposes beginning with 5 minutes, gradually progressing to 10 minutes, 15 minutes, 20 minutes, 30 minutes, and 45 minutes. It became apparent that this approach was indeed successful.

Simultaneously, Lisa was seen at the clinic for additional sessions of imitation and modeling. Appropriate sitting, standing, and greeting gestures were practiced. Conversational skills were also developed. She was counseled on grooming and hygiene. Appropriate clothing selection was made. Bobby socks were soon eliminated from her attire. Lisa began to develop social skills that were socially acceptable and personally gratifying. Through positive channels, she now received the attention she sought.

In addition to working with Lisa, Mrs. C. was counseled on the issues of sterilization, and alternative methods of contraception. In the course of these counseling sessions and instructional endeavors with Lisa, their home life improved. Mark began returning to his classes. "Embarrassing" social situations decreased, and the family seemed to develop a greater appreciation of Lisa's need for attention and the social skills necessary for social acceptability.

This first case illustrated:

1. how one family member can affect the behaviors of other members of the family
2. an assessment process involving the individual, parent, and teacher
3. the use of social learning approach in modifying social behaviors
4. parental counseling
5. normalization principle
6. the use of preventive approach in teaching contraceptive measures

**Case 2**   Marilyn is a 16-year-old moderate to mildly developmentally disabled female. She was initially referred to the clinic for a re-evaluation of her educational needs and counseling toward the choice of a vocation. Upon the completion of the educational evaluation, she was referred by the resident physician for sexual counseling primarily as a preventive measure.

Marilyn was seen at the clinic together with her mother, Mrs. B. They appeared to have a fairly warm relationship. Marilyn was neatly groomed and wore clothing typical for a 16-year-old. Because there were no immediate concerns or problem areas, the preventive approach was used. Sexual counseling and education began with a review of what Marilyn observed as overt physical differences of males and females, their play differences, work differences, etc. Later, Marilyn participated in a co-ed group of teenagers with similar interests, psychosexual maturation, and intellectual abilities.

Group discussions included the following topics: 1) kids at school and how they got along, 2) parents and their restrictions, 3) beginning independence and demand for more responsibilities, 4) selection of opposite sex as a special friend, 5) dating behaviors such as necking and petting, 6) erogenous zones and feelings, 7) what to do when approached by strangers, 8) leaving "unsafe" situations, 9) cultural and moral values, and 10) contraception.

After a period of counseling and education, a reassessment of Marilyn's potential was completed. At that time, Marilyn expressed her desire to one day marry and have children like all other mommies. She had developed many social skills and demonstrated her ability to assume household responsibilities including cooking, laundry, and cleaning house. The care of small children seemed to be another area in which she needed experience. She was assigned to work part-time at the YWCA Nursery Department. Counseling sessions continued to focus on some of the needs of children such as physical, emotional, and intellectual needs as well as the difference between the role of mother and woman including the fact that not all women become "mommies."

This second case illustrates:

1. an assessment of the individual more than the parent primarily because the individual is closer to the normal intellectual level and exhibits greater need for independence
2. the use of preventive approach in teaching
3. utilization of group discussion when appropriate
4. continued reassessment of Marilyn's potential
5. counseling on realistic expectation such as in the situation of marriage and family


## CONCLUSION

The adolescent who is developmentally disabled needs the guidance and counseling necessary to assist him in achieving an optimal living experience in today's complex society. This is of particular importance as the trend continues toward residing in the community setting rather than within institutions.

As health professionals and educators, nurses must be cognizant of the needs of the developmentally disabled adolescent as a person with feelings, hopes, and disappointments who has a desire to achieve personal satisfaction and self-esteem, and the problematic decisions which must be faced by his family and himself.

Certainly, a comprehensive sex education program is a necessary component of any rehabilitation effort for the developmentally disabled. In addition to providing basic sexual and anatomical information, such programs should provide training for professional and nonprofessional staff to deal with various types of activities within the institutional setting, as well as training for families in the home environment and the community. A planned program of social learning situations will help develop appropriate sexual role behavior for all levels of developmental disabilities. Sex education should not be confined solely to the educational facility. It is a concern for all professionals who come in contact with developmentally disabled adolescents.

## SUGGESTED READINGS

Bass, M., and Gelof, M. (eds.). 1972. Sexual Rights and Responsibilities of the Mentally Retarded. Proceedings of the Conference of the American Association on Mental Deficiency, Region 1+. University of Delaware, Newark, Delaware.

Bloom, J. 1969. Sex education for handicapped adolescent. J. School Health. 39(6):363–367.

Fischer, H., and Krajicek, M. 1974. Sexual development of the moderately retarded child: Level of information and parental attitudes. Ment. Retard. 12(3):28–30.

Fischer, H. L., Krajicek, M. J., and Borthick, W. A. 1974. Sex Education for the Developmentally Disabled: A Guide for Parents, Teachers, and Professionals. University Park Press, Baltimore.

Goodman, L., Budner, S., and Lesh, B. 1971. The parents role in sex education for the retarded. Ment. Retard. 9(1) pp. 43–45.

Hall, J. E., Morris, H. L., and Barker, H. R. 1973. Sexual knowledge and attitudes of mentally retarded adolescents. Am. J. Ment. Defic. 77(6):706–709.

Hall, J. E., and Morris, H. L. 1976. Sexual knowledge and attitudes of institutionalized retarded adolescents. Am. J. Ment. Defic. 80(4):382–387.

Hammar, S. L., and Barnard, K. E. 1966. The mentally retarded adolescent. Pediatrics 38(5):845–857.

Hammar, S. L., Wright, L. S. and Jensen, D. L. 1967. Sex Education for the Retarded Adolescent. Clin. Pediatr. 6(11):621–627.

Hutt, M., and Gibby, R. 1976. The Mentally Retarded Child. Allyn and Bacon, Boston.

Johnson, W., Sex education and the mentally retarded. 1969. J. Sex Res. 5(3):179–185.

Kempton, W. and Forman, R. 1976. Guidelines for Training in Sexuality and the Mentally Handicapped. Planned Parenthood Association of Southeastern Pennsylvania, Philadelphia.

Kindred, M., Cohen, J., Penrod, D. and Shaffer, T. (eds.). 1976. The Mentally Retarded Citizen and the Law. Sponsored by the Presidents Committee on Mental Retardation. The Free Press, New York.

Meyerowitz, J. 1971. Sex and the mentally retarded. Med. Aspects Human Sexual. 5(11)95–118.

Mossier, H. D. and Grossman, H. J. 1962. Secondary sex development in mentally deficient individuals. Child Dev. 33:273–286.

Murray, R., and Zentner, J. 1975. Nursing Assessment and Health Promotion Through the Life Span, Prentice-Hall, Englewood Cliffs, N.J.

Pattulo, A. 1969. Puberty in the Girl who is Retarded. National Association for Retarded Children, Arlington, Tex.

Pattulo, A. 1975. The Socio-Sexual Development of the Handicapped Child. Nursing Clin. N. Am. 10(2):361–372.

Whitecraft, C., and Jones, J. 1974. A survey of attitudes about sterilization of retardates. Ment. Retard. 12(1):30–33.

# chapter twelve

# THE PATH TO ADULTHOOD
## Adolescence, Disability, and the Law

Bertram Robert Cottine, J.D.

The law begins to extend new rights and impose new obligations in the midst of the adolescent's rapid physical and emotional development. However, these rights and obligations do not arise at any magic age. Instead the law governs the adolescent's behavior in terms of his or her increased contact with adult society. These include contacts with institutions such as schools and new life situations such as employment. The adolescent may also confront the legal problems which arise from interpersonal relations, as in the case of marriage. While states mark the end of adolescence by setting an age of majority, even this established age may vary according to the legal situation. Majority is also affected by the mental capacity of the person in certain circumstances. With all these variations, it is best to trace the adolescent's progress toward independence in terms of special rights and responsibilities.

If we look at adolescence as progressive preparation for adulthood, there are three major legal problems involving the developmentally disabled which the nurse should be alert to in her practice. The first involves the delivery of special treatment, services, and habilitation for the developmentally disabled. The second legal problem involves the adolescent's right to a free, appropriate public education. The final legal problem to be discussed here is employment. The resolution of this problem is essential to the financial support which is necessary for the sustained independence of the developmentally disabled person.

It is important first to understand the nurse's potential role in the resolution of these legal problems before addressing them specifically.

## PREVENTIVE ADVOCACY AND THE NURSE

The developmentally disabled person confronts a series of legal problems over the course of his or her entire life span. Thus, nurse-advocates must effectively deal with the entire life span of the developmentally disabled person and not simply react to isolated crises whenever they arise. The analogy to preventive medicine is obvious. However, the necessity for preventive advocacy has been almost universally overlooked, particularly the potential partnership between the legal and health professionals. This partnership is based on the health professional's regular contact with the adolescent and the legal professional's capacity to enforce rights and resolve legal problems.

Without effective communication between legal and health professionals, the legal problems of the adolescent may grow to crisis proportions before advocacy is finally provided. This delay may foreclose or significantly restrict the possible alternatives, particularly when education rights are involved. Moreover, delay frequently intensifies the need for services, treatment, and habilitation. As a result, the total demand on these services is increased and their availability is further limited. In addition, the nurse-advocate cannot overlook the fact that adolescents perceive time passing far more slowly than an adult.[1] Finally, the adolescent may not receive legally-entitled services before critical developmental stages have passed. Therefore, any delay in obtaining advocacy services must be avoided.

In preventive and crisis advocacy, the nurse may be involved directly as a nonlegal advocate for the developmentally disabled adolescent. Indirectly, the nurse may be involved as a counselor to the adolescent or an expert witness in a legal proceeding. Parents or guardians, and in some cases, prospective parents, should receive early advice regarding the legal rights of their developmentally disabled child or ward. For example, where amniocentesis reveals a fetus with trisomy 21 (Down's syndrome), the prospective parents should be carefully and compassionately advised regarding the legal options available to them and their child after birth. Moreover, this prenatal period provides an opportunity to consider abortion.[2] In this case, the nurse is in a strategic relationship with the parents to assume both an advocacy and counseling role in identifying legal rights.

Of course, crisis advocacy to meet immediate legal problems is unavoidable because no person's life is completely predictable, even in an institution. However, repetitive crisis intervention over the lifetime of a developmentally disabled person indicates the serious need for preventive advocacy. It is not enough to counsel parents on the medical and psychological situations their child will encounter during adolescence without also identifying the critical legal and human rights which must be implemented during this time. Nor is it enough to intervene with advocacy services to meet a crisis and then abandon the adolescent, only to have the person return again when another crisis arises. This is not to suggest that advocacy should foster the client's dependence. Rather, focus should be on preventive advocacy supported by immediate crisis advocacy only when necessary. Nurse-advocates, like other service providers, should develop a counseling strategy and advocacy plan well in advance of crisis situations.

Nurse-advocates must also be active in the process of deinstitutionalization. First, parents or guardians should be provided appropriate advice on the decision to institutionalize a child. This is extremely important when the conditions at a particular institution have been found to be unconstitutional. Beyond this effort, nurse-advocates should be involved in enforcing the judicially and statutorily created rights within an institution as well as the right to deinstitutionalization. However, once the adolescent has been released he must not be abandoned. Preventive advocacy should precede the release and advocacy services must be provided as the developmentally disabled person progresses to his highest level of independence. In this ongoing relation, nurse-advocates should seek to obtain appropriate community resources for each person through the effective implementation of his legal rights.

Finally, preventive advocacy is particularly important with respect to educational rights because the realization of the child's intellectual, emotional, and social potentials is seriously affected by the schools. Recent federal court decisions have enforced the right to education where the state makes these services generally available.[3] Moreover, Congress recently enacted the Education for All Handicapped Children Act of 1975 which establishes the child's right to a free, appropriate education at public expense. This education must be in the least restrictive setting and it must be made available to all children between the ages of 3 and 18 years by 1978 and the ages of 3 and 21 years by 1980.[4] The early onset of the right to education under this law makes the need for preventive advocacy obvious. However, the extension of educational services beyond the usual school age makes preventive advocacy equally important to the late adolescent.

## DEVELOPMENTALLY DISABLED ASSISTANCE AND BILL OF RIGHTS

### Defining "Developmental Disability"

In 1963, President John F. Kennedy added new momentum to the efforts to protect the human rights of the mentally retarded through the development of specialized evaluation and treatment centers.[5] In 1970, Congress extended this program to persons with epilepsy and cerebral palsy through its definition of "developmental disability."[6] Once again Congress expanded the definition in 1975 (italicized conditions indicate these most recent additions):

1. mental retardation
2. cerebral palsy
3. epilepsy
4. *autism*
5. any other condition closely related to mental retardation which:
   a. results in similar impairment of general intellectual functioning or adaptive behavior, or
   b. requires similar treatment and services; and
6. *dyslexia associated with any of the above conditions*[7]

There are three additional qualifications which must be met on an individual basis. First, the disability must originate before the person is eighteen years old. Second, it must continue or be expected to continue indefinitely. Third, the disability must "constitute a substantial handicap to the person's ability to function normally in society."[8]

Some service providers have attempted to add a fourth qualification based on whether or not the listed condition is the "primary" disability. This limitation is *not* authorized by the statute whatever its usefulness may be in the diagnostic process. For example, before autism was considered a developmental disability, providers denied services to an autistic child who was mentally retarded because the mental retardation was considered "secondary" to the autism. (The autism was considered "primary.")[9] This classification technique demonstrates the need to carefully scrutinize any qualification for services which is not specifically established by the law.

## Bill of Rights

The 1975 Developmentally Disabled Assistance and Bill of Rights Act builds on the numerous court cases which declared unconstitutional the inhuman conditions at institutional and residential facilities for the mentally retarded throughout the United States.[10] Section 111 of the Act removes any lingering doubt about the constitutional rights of the developmentally disabled. Rights which had previously been enforced only by separate judicial orders may now be applied with equal force throughout our nation under this law. Developmentally disabled persons need not await a judicial opinion in their state or federal courts to determine their legal rights.

Section 111 of the Act provides that ". . . persons with developmental disabilities have a right to appropriate treatment, services and habilitation."[11] These services must be designed to maximize the developmental potential of the person. Furthermore, the delivery of these services must be in the setting which is the least restrictive of the person's liberty.[12] This implements the Congressional policy of deinstitutionalization. Moreover, section 111 has extended these rights to noninstitutionalized as well as institutionalized persons.[13] This extension is critical as the process of deinstitutionalization frees developmentally disabled persons to live their lives in the mainstream of our society.

To enforce this right, Congress required the federal and state governments to withhold public funds whenever programs fail to meet certain basic human conditions.

First, Congress required these programs to provide treatment, services and habilitation which is *appropriate* to the developmentally disabled person's needs.[14]

Second, these institutions must meet certain minimum standards to qualify for federal and state funds. While these standards appear to be obvious, the recent litigation involving institutional care facilities makes it all too clear that these rights have been blindly and regularly sacrificed to bureaucratic expedience and callous indifference. A mere listing suffices to identify these most basic human rights. However, each word in the statute should be read with special care for it reveals shameful events in the history of our institutions for the developmentally disabled:

1.  nourishing, well balanced daily diet
2.  appropriate and sufficient medical and dental service
3.  prohibition of physical restraint unless absolutely necessary
4.  prohibition of excessive chemical restraint
5.  visitation by close relatives at reasonable hours without prior notice
6.  adequate safety and fire standards as established by the Secretary (HEW)[15]

Items 3 and 4 require elaboration. Neither physical restraint nor excessive chemical restraint may be used as a punishment or as a substitute for habilitation. Moreover, chemical restraints must not interfere with the statutorily guaranteed right to treatment, services, and habilitation.

Further, all programs for the developmentally disabled should meet "standards . . . designed to assure the most favorable possible outcome."[16] This includes nonresidential as well as residential programs.

In section 112 of the Act, Congress recognized that the right to treatment, services, and habilitation requires affirmative efforts to programmatically plan and deliver services for each developmentally disabled person.[17] As a result, section 112 requires a written individualized habilitation plan for each person who receives services from a program funded from the state allotment. It is here that the statutory bill of rights in section 111 and the advocacy and counseling services of section 113 emerge in a concrete strategy for delivering services. Implementation of statutory and constitutional rights under section 112 requires careful attention to the *details of the proposed program* and the *actual delivery of the identified services.*[18]

The habilitation plan must be developed jointly by a representative of the program and the developmentally disabled person. Where appropriate, the parent, guardian, or another representative may also participate.[19] The plan must include:

1.  long range habilitation goals
2.  intermediate habilitation objectives facilitating these goals
3.  statement of specific services to be provided and personnel required
4.  dates for the initiation of services and their duration[20]

Annual review of the plan is mandatory. The participatory rights of the developmentally disabled person and the parent, guardian, or other representative must be preserved in this review.

Advocacy is crucial to the development of a habilitation plan. It should focus on the client's evaluation of the possible options in habilitation, the recognition of their potential impact, and the appropriate development and finalization of the habilitation plan. These advocacy efforts involve the annual review of its actual implementation as well as its initial development.[21]

## EDUCATION

In 1975 there were eight million handicapped children and youth in the United States. More than one-half of these persons did not receive appropriate educational services which would enable them to enjoy full equality of educational opportunity; one million were excluded entirely from the public school system. In addition to children with identified handicaps, many other children have handicaps which have gone undetected. In response to this pressing need, Congress authorized financial support to assist state and local educational agencies to assume their responsibility in providing education for all handicapped children.[22]

As a condition to this financial assistance, all handicapped children must be provided a free, appropriate education which emphasizes special education and related services designed to meet their unique needs.[23] This right extends to children between 3 and 18 years of age by September 1, 1978 and to children and adults between 3 and 21 years of age by September 1, 1980.[24] The state must not only serve those children who have asserted their right to a free appropriate public education, it must conduct an extensive "child find" effort. This identification and evaluation is crucial to implementing the right to education.

The right to a free, appropriate public education includes four components. The education must:

1. be provided at public expense
2. meet state educational standards
3. include preschool, elementary, and secondary education
4. be based on an "individualized education program"[25]

This last requirement parallels the provision for an individualized habilitation plan in section 112 of the Developmentally Disabled

Assistance and Bill of Rights Act of 1975. Under Public Law 94-142 the individualized education program must be a *written* statement containing:

1.  present levels of educational performance
2.  annual goals including short term instructional objectives
3.  an identification of specific educational services to be delivered
4.  extent of participation in regular educational programs
5.  appropriate objective criteria and evaluation procedures[26]

There are three other important aspects of the right to a free, appropriate public education. First, children with handicaps are to be educated with children who are not handicapped.[27] There is only one extremely limited exception. Special classes, separate schooling, and other removal from the regular educational environment may occur only when education in a regular class cannot be satisfactorily achieved even with the use of supplementary aids and services.[28] Second, where a child has been referred to or placed in a private facility by a state or local agency, the placement must be at no cost to the parents.[29] In addition, a private facility which accepts referrals or placements must provide the child with the same rights accorded the child under this Act in a public facility.[30] Third, the testing and evaluation materials used by educational agencies must be selected and administered to eliminate racial or cultural discrimination.[31]

None of these rights to a free, appropriate public education is secure without procedural safeguards. Two of these protections have special significance to the nurse dealing with developmentally disabled adolescents. Where the adolescent has not been accurately or thoroughly evaluated by the educational agency, the child has a right to an *independent* educational evaluation at no expense.[32] Nurses should carefully examine the evaluations performed by the education agency. Where appropriate, they should suggest that the parents or child exercise the right to an independent evaluation. In addition, the nurse must be aware of the child's right to be represented by an attorney or an individual with special knowledge or training with respect to handicapped children.[33] Thus, nurses familiar with developmental disabilities may serve as advocates for the adolescent's right to a free, appropriate public education.

## EMPLOYMENT

The final key to the developmentally disabled adolescent's independence is self-sustaining employment. A nurse-advocate can assist in the implementation of the adolescent's rights to treatment and education and yet ultimately fail if these services do not yield an employment payoff.

The employment relation is a complex series of legal events which occur over a considerable period of time. These events take on special significance for the developmentally disabled person seeking his first job. Of course, the most critical event is hiring. This includes the employer's formulation of a job description with its specific qualifications as well as the process of application, interviewing, and placement.

The state and federal governments regulate the hiring of handicapped persons through a number of legal mechanisms. On a state level, fair employment practices laws prohibit discrimination against handicapped persons. However, each state has developed its own approach to these problems. Thus, the solutions vary widely. In some states, their general civil rights laws include handicapped persons as a protected class of individuals. In other cases, the states have paralleled the federal approach by developing separate protections. (The most recent compilation of state laws is contained in the Appendix at the end of this chapter.)

The conduct which is considered "discriminatory" will vary according to the particular law applied. In addition, more than one law may apply to a particular situation. For example, an employer's refusal to hire a developmentally disabled person merely because of his or her disability may be illegal under both state and federal laws. Furthermore, there are two general types of employment discrimination laws. The first type of law prohibits discriminatory activity by the employer against handicapped individuals who apply for a job or seek advancement.[34] The second requires "affirmative action," usually in the form of an "affirmative action plan," which the employer must develop and follow in the employment and advancement of handicapped persons.[35]

Specific discriminatory activity regulated under a single law is usually further defined by the administrative agency which is charged with enforcing the law. These more detailed definitions usually take the form of regulations or guidelines. No understanding of the statutory law is accurate without reference to the most recent version of these regulations or guidelines.

On a federal level there are three important pieces of legislation to protect handicapped persons in their search for employment. The first is the Rehabilitation Act of 1973, specifically sections 501, 503, and 504.[36]

Section 501 establishes an Interagency Committee on Handicapped Employees to review regularly the adequacy of hiring, placement, and advancement practices with respect to federal government employees who are handicapped. Each federal agency is required to develop an *affirmative action program plan* which must be reviewed and approved by the U.S. Civil Service Commission. This plan must include sufficient assurances, procedures and commitments to provide adequate hiring, placement, and advancement opportunities for handicapped individuals. Handicapped individuals who are employed by a federal agency must consult their particular agency's plan to determine their specific rights and the procedure for protecting them. The gap between written affirmative action plans and actual federal agency practice is currently under critical study.[37]

Section 503 is directed toward discrimination by employers who have contracts with the federal government in excess of $2,500.[38] The important key to coverage under this section is a *contract* with a federal department or agency. This contract must be ". . . for the procurement of personal property and nonpersonal services (including construction) for the United States . . ."[39]

Section 503 parallels section 501 in requiring each contractor ". . . to take affirmative action to employ and advance in employment qualified handicapped individuals . . ." in *all* departments of the employer's business. If the contractor has failed to comply with: (1) his own affirmative action plan or (2) the requirements of section 503 and the implementing regulations, then the handicapped individual involved may file a complaint with the Office of Federal Contract Compliance Programs (OFCCP) in the U.S. Department of Labor.[40] In acting on a valid complaint, the Labor Department may take appropriate action against the employer. This action might include back wages where a disabled person proves that he was not hired because of his disability.

Section 504 of the Rehabilitation Act states that no program or activity which receives Federal financial assistance may exclude from participation, deny benefits, or discriminate against any otherwise qualified handicapped individual.[41] This section has a vast impact far beyond the programs and activities which have been specifically developed for handicapped individuals. For example, section 504 has been used to challenge federally assisted mass transit systems which failed to purchase accessible buses.[42]

Similarly, section 106 of the Developmentally Disabled Assistance and Bill of Rights Act of 1975,[43] and section 606 of the

Education for All Handicapped Children Act of 1975,[44] require the
recipients of funds under either Act ". . . to employ and advance in
employment qualified handicapped individuals . . ."[43]

These two affirmative action provisions apply equally to state as
well as private service providers which receive federal funds. The
reason for these Congressional requirements is clear. The exclusion of
handicapped persons from employment with these programs is fundamentally inconsistent with the social purpose underlying these laws.
Exclusion also deprives these programs of the perspective of
employees whose personal experiences will sensitize the programs to
the problems of the disabled.

Finally, the nurse should not overlook the special job training and
placement opportunities which are available in vocational rehabilitation programs. These opportunities are particularly important when
the adolescent is: (1) no longer attending class, or (2) awaiting disposi-
tion of a juvenile charge against him.


## CONCLUSION

The legal rights of the developmentally disabled are constantly emerging as the judicial and legislative processes identify rights which are
critical to the full integration of the developmentally disabled into our
society. The goal is to maximize their abilities and minimize their
disabilities. However, we cannot leave disabled persons without effective advocates in our increasingly complex society. At stake is our
constitutional promise and human belief that the real strength of our
society is built on our shared abilities and not our everpresent frailties
and disabilities. Furthermore, whenever the fabric of one person's life
is torn by discrimination, inaction or indifference then all our lives are
diminished. The nurse-advocate has a vital role to play in protecting
the rights of the developmentally disabled adolescent.


## NOTES

1. J. Goldstein et al. 1973. *Beyond the Best Interests of The Child.*
   (*passim*).
2. *Roe v. Wade*, 410 U.S. 113 (1973).
3. E.g., *Mills v. D.C. Board of Education*, 348 F. Supp. 866 (D.D.C. 1972).
4. Pub. L. 94-142, § 5(a), 89 Stat. 780–781, *amending* Education of the
   Handicapped Act of 1970, 84 Stat. 175 (codified as 20 U.S.C. §§ 1401
   *et seq.*)
5. Mental Retardation Facilities and Community Health Centers
   Construction Act of 1963, Pub. L. 88-164, 77 Stat. 282.

6. Developmental Disabilities Services and Facilities Construction Amendments of 1970, Pub. L. 91-517, § 102(b), 84 Stat. 1325, *amending* 42 U.S.C. § 2691 (1970).
7. Developmentally Disabled Assistance and Bill of Rights Act of 1975, Pub. L. 94-103, § 125, 89 Stat. 497, *amending* 42 U.S.C. § 6001(7).
8. 42 U.S.C. § 6001(7)(B)–(D).
9. Hearings on S.3378: Developmentally Disabled Assistance and Bill of Rights Act of 1974 Before Subcomm. on the Handicapped of the Senate Comm. on Labor and Public Welfare, 93d Cong., 2d Sess., 408–430 (1974).
10. The seminal case involves the Partlow State School in Alabama, *Wyatt v. Hardin*, 325 F. Supp. 781 (M.D. Ala. 1971), 344 F. Supp. 1341 (1971), 314 F. Supp. 373, (1972), *aff'd in part, modified in part sub nom. Wyatt v. Aderholt*, 503 F.2d 1305 (5th Cir. 1974).
11. 42 U.S.C. § 6010(1).
12. 42 U.S.C. § 6010(2).
13. 42 U.S.C. §§ 6010(1), (2), (4).
14. 42 U.S.C. §§ 6010(1), (3)(A).
15. 42 U.S.C. §§ 6010(3)(B)(i)–(vi).
16. 42 U.S.C. § 6010(4).
17. 42 U.S.C. § 6011.
18. *Id.*
19. 42 U.S.C. § 6011(b)(2).
20. 42 U.S.C. § 6011(b)(3)–(4).
21. 42 U.S.C. § 6011(a)(2), (c).
22. Education of All Handicapped Children Act of 1975, Pub. L. 94-142, § 3(a), 89 Stat. 774–775, *amending* Education of the Handicapped Act, § 601, 84 Stat. 179 (1970).
23. 20 U.S.C. § 1412(1).
24. 20 U.S.C. § 1412(2)(B).
25. 20 U.S.C. § 1401(18).
26. 20 U.S.C. §§ 1401(19), 1414(a)(5).
27. 20 U.S.C. § 1412(5)(B).
28. *Id.*
29. 20 U.S.C. § 1413(a)(4)(B)(i).
30. 20 U.S.C. § 1413(a)(4)(B)(ii).
31. 20 U.S.C. § 1412(5)(c).
32. 20 U.S.C. § 1415(b)(1)(A).
33. 20 U.S.C. § 1415(d).
34. 29 U.S.C. § 793.
35. 29 U.S.C. § 794.
36. 29 U.S.C. §§ 791, 793–794.
37. This study is being conducted by the Disability Rights Center, 1346 Connecticut Avenue, N.W., Washington, D.C. 20036, under the direction of Deborah Kaplan, Esq.
38. 29 U.S.C. § 793.
39. *Id.*
40. Contact the regional office of the U.S. Dept. of Labor for the address and phone number of the OFCCP covering your area.

41.  29 U.S.C. § 794.
42.  *Snowden v. Birmingham-Jefferson County Transit Authority*, Civ. No. 75-G-330-S (N.D. Ala., June 23, 1975), *appeal docketed*, No. 75-3411 (5th Cir., August 10, 1975).
43.  42 U.S.C. § 6005.
44.  20 U.S.C. § 1405.

## SUGGESTED READINGS

Brakel, S., and Rock, R. (eds.). 1971. The Mentally Disabled and the Law. American Bar Foundation, Chicago.

Commission on the Mentally Disabled, American Bar Association. Mental Disability Law Reporter (periodical).

Ennis, D., and Friedman, P. (eds.). 1973. Legal Rights of the Mentally Handicapped. Practising Law Institute, New York.

Friedman, P. (ed.). 1976. The Rights of the Mentally Retarded. American Civil Liberties Union, New York.

Kindred, M. et al (eds.). 1976. The Mentally Retarded Citizen and the Law. President's Commission on Mental Retardation, Washington, D.C.

President's Committee on Employment of the Handicapped. 1976. A Handbook on the Legal Rights of Handicapped People. Washington, D.C.

Stone, A. 1975. Mental Health and Law: A System in Transition. National Institute of Mental Health, Washington, D.C.

## APPENDIX: STATE STATUTES REGARDING EMPLOYMENT[a]

FEPC—A Fair Employment Practices Commission is a body established by statute to investigate, review, and resolve complaints of discrimination in hiring, dismissal, and terms and conditions of employment.[b]

HRC—A Human Rights Commission (or Civil Rights Commission) is a body established by statute to investigate, review, and resolve complaints of unlawful discrimination in housing, public accommodations, education, employment, and other areas.[b]

EOL—An Equal Opportunity Law is a civil rights statute which may or may not provide for administrative enforcement, a criminal penalty, or a private cause of action.

CS—A Civil Service statute is a law which affects only all or part of those persons employed by the state civil service system. Some states which do not have a statute prohibiting discrimination do have an administrative policy to that effect.

WCL—A White Cane Law is a statute designed primarily to define the rights and responsibilities of blind persons, particularly in relation to the use of white canes and guide dogs. In some states, it has been broadened to include other handicapped persons as well.

CP—A Criminal Penalty is provided in some states, either for the initial discrimination or for violation of an order of a Fair Employment Practices Commission or a Human Rights Commission.

PS—A Policy Statement is a statute which says that nondiscrimination is the official policy of the state, but provides no enforcement mechanism.

COA—A Cause of Action is the right of an aggrieved person to bring a lawsuit for unlawful discrimination, either as an exclusive remedy or in addition to an administrative remedy.

[a] Reprinted from National Center for Law and the Handicapped, State Statutes Regarding Employment, *Amicus* 1:30-35, 1976.
[b] Decisions by these Commissions are always reviewable by the courts as well. Such a review would take place after one of the parties involved in the complaint would appeal the agency's decision.

| State | Type of statute | Citation |
|---|---|---|
| Alabama | CS | Alabama Code Title 55, Section 307(1) |
| | WCL | Alabama Code 3, Section 6(1); 36, Section 58(53) |
| Alaska | HRC | Alaska Statute Section 18.80.010 to Section 18.80.300 |
| | CP | Alaska Stat. Section 18.80.270 |
| | COA | Alaska Stat. Section 18.80.145, Section 22.10.020(c) |
| | WCL, PS | Alaska Stat. Section 18.06.010 et seq. |
| Arizona | WCL | Arizona Revised Statute Section 24-411, Section 28-798, Section 34-402 et seq. |
| Arkansas | WCL | Ark. Stat. Section 75-631 and 632, Section 78-211 et seq. Ark. Stat. Section 82-2901 |
| California | FEPC | Calif. Labor Code Section 1410 to Section 1433 |
| | CP | Calif. Labor Code Section 1430 |
| | WCL | Calif. Labor Code Pt. 2.5, Section 54 to Section 54.6 |
| | | Calif. Penal Code Section 643, Section 643(a), Section 643(b) |
| | PS | Calif. Gov't Code Section 3550 |
| | | Calif. Labor Code Section 1411 |
| Colorado | WCL | Colo. Rev. Stat. Section 18-13-107 |
| | PS | Colo. Rev. Stat. Section 24-34-801 |
| Connecticut | HRC | Conn. Gen. Stat. Section 31-122 to Section 31-128 |
| | WCL | Conn. Gen. Stat. Section 53-211 |
| Delaware | WCL | Del. Code Tit. 16, Chap. 95 |
| | | Del. Code Tit. 21, Section 2144 and Section 2150 |
| | PS | Del. Code Tit. 16, Section 9501 |
| District of Columbia | HRC | D.C. Title 34 (Human Rights Law), Chap. 11 and 29 |
| | CP | D.C. Code Encyclopedia Section 6-1501, Tit. 34, Section 35.1(b) |
| | COA | D.C. Tit. 34, Section 35.2 |
| | WCL, PS | D.C. Code Ency. Section 6-1501 et seq. |
| | CS | D.C. Code Ency. Section 6-1504 |
| Florida | WCL, PS | Fla. Stat. Section 413.08 |
| | CP | Fla. Stat. Section 413.08(5) |

*Continued*

| State | Type of statute | Citation |
|---|---|---|
| Georgia | CS | Ga. Code Section 40-2201 |
| | WCL | Ga. Code Section 79-601, Section 79-9901 |
| Hawaii | FEPC | Hawaii Rev. Stat. Section 378-1 to Section 378-10 |
| | CP | Hawaii Rev. Stat. Section 378-10 |
| | CS | Hawaii Rev. Stat. Section 76-1 |
| | WCL, PS | Hawaii Rev. Stat. Section 347-1 *et seq.* |
| Idaho | HRC | House Bill 336, amending Idaho Code Section 67-5901 *et seq.* |
| | CS | Idaho Code Section 56-707, Section 59-1025 |
| | WCL | Idaho Code Section 56-701 *et seq.*, Section 18-5810 to Section 18-5812 |
| | PS | Idaho Code Section 56-701 |
| Illinois | EOL | Ill. Rev. Stat. Chap. 38, Section 65-21 *et seq.* |
| | FEPC | Ill. Rev. Stat. Chap. 48, Section 851 *et seq.* |
| | WCL | Ill. Rev. Stat. Chap. 23, Section 3361 *et seq.* |
| Indiana | HRC | Ind. Code Section 22-9-1-4 |
| | WCL | Ind. Stat. Section 10-4925 to Section 10-4927 |
| | | Ind. Code Section 35-29-6-1 |
| | PS | Ind. Code Section 16-7-5-1 |
| Iowa | HRC | Iowa Code Section 601A.1 to Section 601A.17 |
| | WCL | Iowa Code Section 321.332 to Section 321.334 |
| | PS | Iowa Code Section 601D.1 |
| Kansas | HRC | Kan. Stat. Section 44-1001 to Section 44-1038 |
| | CP | Kan. Stat. Section 44-1013 |
| | WCL | Kan. Stat. Section 8-1542 |
| | PS | Kan. Stat. Section 39–1101 |
| Kentucky | EOL | House Bill 407 (1976) |
| | COA | House Bill 407 (1976), Section 12 |
| | CP | House Bill 407 (1976), Section 13 |
| | WCL | Ky. Rev. Stat. Section 189.575 |
| | HRC | Ky. Rev. Stat., Chap. 207 |
| Louisiana | WCL | La. Rev. Stat. Section 32-217 |
| | PS | La. Rev. Stat. Section 46-1951 |

| State | Type of statute | Citation |
|---|---|---|
| Maine | HRC | Me. Rev. Stat. Section 4551 to Section 4613 |
|  | COA | Me. Rev. Stat. Section 4621 to Section 4623 |
|  | WCL, PS | Me. Tit. 17, Section 1311 *et seq.* |
| Maryland | HRC | Md. Code Art. 49B, Section 1 to Section 20 |
|  | CS | Md. Code Art. 64A, Section 12 |
|  | WCL | Md. Code Art. 66½, Section 194 |
|  | PS | Md. Code Art. 30, Section 33 |
| Massachusetts | FEPC, CP | Laws of Mass., Chap 149, Section 24K |
|  | WCL | Mass. Chap. 90, Section 14A |
| Michigan | HRC | Senate Bill No. 749 (effective 3/30/77) |
|  | WCL | Mich. Stat. Section 28.770(1) *et seq.* |
| Minnesota | HRC | Minn. Stat. Section 363.01 to Section 363.14 |
|  | CP | Minn. Stat. Section 363.101 |
|  | COA | Minn. Stat. Section 363.14 |
|  | CS | Minn. Gov't Code of Fair Practice, 9/1/73 |
|  | WCL | Minn. Stat. Section 169.202 |
|  | PS | Minn. Stat. Section 363.12, Section 256C.01 |
| Mississippi | WCL | Miss. Code Section 43-6-1 *et seq.* |
|  | PS | Miss. Code Section 43-6-3 |
| Missouri | WCL | Mo. Stat. Section 304.080 to Section 304.110 |
| Montana | HRC | Mont. Rev. Code Section 64-301 to Section 64-312 |
|  | CP | Mont. Rev. Code Section 64-312 |
|  | COA | Mont. Rev. Code Section 64-329 |
|  | CS | Mont. Rev. Code Section 64-317 |
|  | WCL, PS | Mont. Rev. Code Section 71-1303 *et seq.* |
| Nebrasha | FEPC | Neb. Rev. Stat. Section 48.1101 to Section 48.1125 |
|  | CP | Neb. Rev. Stat. Section 48.1123 |
|  | CS | Neb. Rev. Stat. Section 20.131 |
|  | WCL, PS | Neb. Rev. Stat. Section 20.126 *et seq.*, Section 28.478 to Section 28.480 |
| Nevada | FEPC | Nev. Rev. Stat. Section 613.310 to Section 613.430 |
|  | COA | Nev. Rev. Stat. Section 613.420 |
|  | WCL | Nev. Rev. Stat. Section 426.510 |

*Continued*

| State | Type of statute | Citation |
|-------|-----------------|----------|
| New Hampshire | HRC | N.H. Rev. Stat. Section 354-A:1 to Section 354-A:14 |
|  | CP | N.H. Rev. Stat. Section 354-A:12 |
|  | WCL, PS | N.H. Rev. Stat. Section 167-C *et seq.*, Section 263.58 |
| New Jersey | HRC | N.J. Stat. Section 10:5-1 to Section 10:5-28 |
|  | CP | N.J. Stat. Section 10:5-26 |
|  | WCL | N.J. Stat. Section 10:5-29 and Section 10:5-30 |
| New Mexico | HRC | N.M. Stat. Section 4-33-1 to Section 4-33-13 |
|  | WCL, PS | N.M. Stat. Section 12-26-1 *et seq.* |
| New York | HRC | McKinney's Consolidated Law Chap. 18, Section 15-290 to Section 15-301 |
|  | CP | N.Y. McKinney's Con. Law Section 15-299 |
|  | COA | N.Y. McKinney's Con. Law Section 15-297(9) |
|  | CS | Civil Service Law Section 55 |
|  | WCL | Vehicle & Traffic Law Section 1153 |
| North Carolina | CS | N.C. Gen. Stat. Section 128-15.3 |
|  | WCL | N.C. Gen. Stat. Section 20-175.1 *et seq.* |
|  | PS | N.C. Gen. Stat. Section 168-1 *et seq.* |
| North Dakota | WCL, PS | N.D. Centennial Code Section 25-13-01 *et seq.* |
| Ohio | HRC | Ohio Rev. Code Section 4112.01 *et seq.* |
|  | CP | Ohio Rev. Code Section 4112.99 |
|  | WCL | Ohio Rev. Code Section 4511.47 |
| Oklahoma | CS | Okl. Stat. Tit. 74, Section 818 |
|  | WCL | Okl. Stat. Tit. 7, Section 11 to Section 13, Section 19.1 and Section 19.2 |
| Oregon | FEPC | Ore. Rev. Stat. Section 659.400 to Section 659.435 |
|  | WCL | Ore. Rev. Stat. Section 346.610, Section 483.214, Section 487.3 |
|  | PS | Ore. Rev. Stat. Section 659.405 |
| Pennsylvania | HRC | Pa. Stat. Tit. 43, Section 951 to Section 963 |
|  | CP | Pa. State. Tit. 43, Section 961 |
|  | COA | Pa. Stat. Tit. 43, Section 962(c) |
|  | WCL | Pa. Stat. Tit. 75, Section 1039 |

| State | Type of statute | Citation |
|-------|-----------------|----------|
| Rhode Island | HRC | R.I. Gen. Laws Section 28-5-1 to Section 28-5-39 |
| | WCL | R.I. Gen. Laws Section 31-18-3 to Section 31-18-16 |
| | PS | R.I. Gen. Laws Section 25-2-13, Section 28-5-3 |
| South Carolina | WCL | S.C. Code Section 46-438 *et seq.*, Section 71-300.51 *et seq.* |
| | CS | S.C. Code Section 71-300.56 |
| South Dakota | WCL | S.D. Laws Section 32-27-6 *et seq.* |
| Tennessee | EOL | Public Chapter No. 457 L. 1976. |
| | WCL | Tenn. Code Section 59-880 and Section 59-881 |
| | PS | Tenn. Code Section 14-627, Section 14-638 |
| Texas | EOL | Vernon's Tex. Civ. Stat. Art. 4419e |
| | CP | Vernon's Tex. Civ. Stat. Art. 4419e, Section 6(a) |
| | COA | Vernon's Tex. Civ. Stat. Art. 4419e, Section 6(b) |
| | WCL | Vernon's Tex. Civ. Stat. Art. 4419e, Art. 6701e |
| Utah | WCL | Utah Code Section 41-6-80.1 |
| | CS | Utah Code Section 26-28-3 |
| | PS | Utah Code Section 26-28-1 |
| Vermont | EOL | Vt. Stat. Tit. 21, Section 498 |
| | COA | Vt. Stat. Tit. 21, Section 498(b) |
| | WCL | Vt. Stat. Tit. 213, Section 1106 |
| Virginia | EOL | Va. Code Section 401.1-28.7 |
| | COA | Va. Code Section 401.1-28.7 |
| | CS | Va. Code Section 63.1-171.6 |
| | WCL | Va. Code Section 63.171.1 *et seq.*, Section 46.1-237 |
| Washington | HRC | Rev. Code Wash. Section 49.60.010 to Section 49.60.330 |
| | CP | Rev. Code Wash. Section 49.60.310 |
| | WCL, PS | Rev. Code Wash. Section 70.84.010 *et seq.* |
| West Virginia | HRC | W. Va. Code Section 5-11-1 to Section 5-11-16 |
| | CP | W. Va. Code Section 5-11-14 |
| | WCL, PS | W. Va. Code Section 5-15-1 *et seq.* |

*Continued*

| State | Type of statute | Citation |
|-------|-----------------|----------|
| Wisconsin | FEPC | Wisc. Stat. Section 111.31 to Section 111.37 |
| | COA | Wisc. Stat. Section 111.36(3)(c) |
| | CS | Wisc. Stat. Section 16.14, Section 63.32 |
| | WCL | Wisc. Stat. Section 346.26 |
| Wyoming | WCL, PS | Wyo. Stat. Section 42-35.1 to Section 42-35.4 |

# chapter thirteen

# TOMORROW
# Toward Fulfillment
# as an Adult

Ann M. Zuzich, R.N., M.S.

The anticipation of adulthood for the person who is developmentally disabled has inherent in it the same sources of anxiety that each human being encounters during periods of transitional development. Successful movement into an adulthood with reasonable expectations for self-actualization can be correlated to life experiences during the preceding developmental stages of the individual's growth. The meaning of self-actualization or self-fulfillment as used in this paper is best described by Maslow, "Self-actualization is defined in various ways but a solid core of agreement is perceptible. All definitions accept or imply: (1) acceptance and expression of the inner core or self, i.e., actualization of these latent capacities and potentialities, "full functioning," availability of the human and personal essence; and (2) minimal presence of ill health, neuroses, and psychosis, of loss or diminution of the basic human and personal capacities." (Maslow, 1962).

The authors of the preceding chapters have addressed themselves to the application of knowledge from many professional disciplines for the promotion of the necessary growth of the developmentally disabled adolescent which will permit such self-actualization to occur.

The developmentally disabled young adult, like his sibling who is not disabled, is primarily concerned with three specific tasks: 1) detachment from parents or parental surrogates in the establishment of identity, 2) vocational choice, and 3) heterosexual activity including consideration of marriage and parenthood.

His capability in the performance of these tasks will, of course, be influenced by his degree of disability and his previous life experiences.

There are additional variables with significant potential for impact on the degree to which the person who is developmentally disabled may progress toward self-actualization or self-fulfillment. These variables must be discussed within the framework of societal development. The important changes which seem immanent in the social structure of the world in which we live, and the professional and personal responsibility to influence those changes demands careful consideration.

Meyer speaks of the behavior of young adults as a reflection of the "changes, problems and opportunities of society as a whole." (Meyer, 1973). It is obvious that the behavior of the developmentally disabled young adult, then, will also reflect societal development.

The degree to which our society can accept the adult who is developmentally disabled as a member of a community with a contribution to make, and with the same rights of all citizens, influences the potential for the young adult to establish his own identity and move toward independence. It is significant that a measurable improvement in public attitudes toward retarded persons is taking place. It has been reported that there are increasing numbers of people who believe that most retarded persons are able to lead independent lives (President's Committee on Mental Retardation, 1976). It has been demonstrated that application of present knowledge makes it possible to reduce the dependency of every retarded person regardless of the degree of disability, and also makes it possible for the majority of retarded people to become fully integrated, self-sufficient adults, no longer stigmatized by the label of "retardation."

However, the stereotypical view of the developmentally disabled person as a burden or as a threat will not diminish in a society where hedonistic values flourish. The move toward humanistic values is the base from which will emerge the public support for the services that the adult who is developmentally disabled must have if he is to achieve some degree of self-fulfillment. It is hopeful, that, despite long years of the rejection of this rather large segment of our population, there has always remained a small minority who persisted in the belief that this population was neither helpless nor hopeless. Finally, that small minority has grown so that their voices are being heard.

Changes are occurring indicating society's awareness that steps can be taken to assure a sufficiency of material goods for all and that men can confidently solve the problems inherent in achieving such a state of sufficiency. Campaigns to eliminate hunger and poverty are being mounted at local, state, national, and international levels, involving many different kinds of approaches. The goal is one toward which we move very slowly; eventual attainment will only come through determination and persistence. The developmentally disabled adult is in a segment of our population especially vulnerable to the affects of poverty, so the success of the efforts to eliminate poverty become particularly important to him.

The debate intensifies about the establishment of criteria for the determination of the existence of the human being. Thoughtful men and women are confronting this issue as well as other social, ethical, and legal issues through organizations established for the purpose of stimulating pertinent scientific inquiry and public education. One such organization is the Institute of Society, Ethics and the Life Sciences, which disseminates many publications that have great potential for influencing public attitudes and decisions. It becomes clear as one reviews these publications that they have serious implications for determining either the dehumanization of the developmentally disabled person or the enhancement of his life. Professional and personal responsibility demands that advocates for the developmentally disabled pursue activity through such groups so that their influence can be felt, as we struggle with conflicting proposals to improve the social climate within which all of us must live.

Basic to the performance of developmental tasks expressing movement toward self-actualization is the maintenance of health. The developmentally disabled adult can minimally expect the same quality of health care that is available for other persons in the community. Demands are being made that the education and training of health care providers include specific information about the developmentally disabled population and supervised clinical experience in their care. The Division of Nursing of the American Association of Mental Deficiency has been particularly concerned about proposing ways to include concepts about the care of this population in basic nursing programs. One very well organized detailed plan was implemented at the University of Tennessee that resulted in modification of the curriculum content to include concepts about the developmentally disabled population in the baccalaureate program for nurses.

The nursing contribution to the development of self-fulfillment in the developmentally disabled adult can be significant. Opportunities abound for teaching about the maintenance of health to developmentally disabled adults as well as to those people who have the responsibility for some degree of supervision of their activities in the community. It has been the experience of this writer that group home operators, agency case managers, foster home parents, and others involved with assisting developmentally disabled adults are hungry for basic knowledge about health maintenance. Practicing nurses must give much more attention to this need.

Increasing numbers of severely and profoundly developmentally disabled adults are residing in nursing homes. The limitations of the care available in many nursing homes has been publicly exposed. Professional nursing associations have been actively involved in working with state legislators, citizen organizations, and members of the Congress to resolve the many problems that contribute to inadequate nursing home care.

As educational programs are modified, recent graduates are better prepared to care for the developmentally disabled population. The largest majority of nurses in practice, however, have not had the opportunity to learn about the developmentally disabled. Occasional, short continuing education programs have been offered by different groups with varying degrees of success. In some states, such as Michigan and California, health occupation licensing acts are being revised to include mandatory continuing education as a condition for re-licensing. It is anticipated that this will provide the motivation for an increased effort in this area.

Community health nurses are particularly suitable to serve as primary health care providers for the developmentally disabled population living in the community. Limited resources often restrict the development of this type of service. Accessibility and availability of generic and special medical services must be more broadly provided. Increasing numbers of advocates for the developmentally disabled are insisting that the quantity and quality of health service be improved. The degree to which that improvement can be achieved is closely related to the success of the attempts to modify the health care delivery system to include an acceptable standard of health care for all citizens.

Financial independence is one of the measures that demonstrate movement toward independence, and financial independence is now within reach for more persons with developmental disability than has ever been true in the past. One of the most common ways of achieving that financial independence is through competitive employment. Increasing numbers of adults who are developmentally disabled are competitively employed, because they have proven that, when given appropriate training, they are capable employees. "They are successfully engaging in jobs such as carpenter, dishwasher, food service worker, animal caretaker, key punch operator, office machine operator, radio repair, telephone operator, ward attendant, vehicle maintenance" (President's Committee on Mental Retardation, 1976). As increasing numbers of developmentally disabled adults are ready for competitive employment, it is imperative that the problems of scarce employment in our society be resolved so that opportunity for employment is available to all. Economic uncertainty can be a mechanism for the denial of opportunity to this vulnerable segment of our society. There is growing awareness, however, that developmentally disabled adults are themselves able to assert their rights through established mechanisms. Local bargaining units with union affiliation, whose members are developmentally disabled, have been organized to negotiate contracts for the mutual interests and benefits of the workers and the employers. The Handicapped Workers Union, Division of Local No. 16, International Union Dolls, Toys, Playthings and Allied Products, AFL-CIO, Chicago, provided information about their organization during the 1976 annual meeting of the American Association of Mental Deficiency, and one of their members was available to answer questions.

When the degree of disability is such that competitive employment is not possible, employment opportunities in sheltered workshops are a viable alternative. A national survey by Suazo, in 1973, revealed that most of the 110 workshops serving the mentally retarded "needed immediate help in many areas, especially in placing clients on jobs, providing financial support to those clients who could not produce at a high enough rate for competitive employment, and providing better training for workshop staff" (President's Committee on Mental Retardation, 1976). There is a pressing need for developing the quantity and quality of this kind of service for the developmentally disabled whose degree of handicap is significant. Even when performance is minimal, and therefore, the reimbursement is limited, the value to the adult justifies the provision of the service, according to some authorities. "Handicapped adults who can work, even if only in a limited way, are more likely to be occupied as adults and treated accordingly than are adults who are totally dependent on others for their subsistence" (Tizard, 1975).

Other methods of providing for many severely handicapped developmentally disabled adults to move toward a kind of financial independence have begun to emerge. One of these is the Supplemental Security Income Program through which the Federal government guaranteed a minimum income to persons with insufficient resources for the first time in 1974. This program has been a significant factor in the development of a variety of choices for different living arrangements for retarded people. The debate about the passing of the Protestant work ethic in our society merits some attention as we view this particular development. Seemingly refuting the position of Tizard, to which there was previous reference, Edgerton and Bercovici reported from a study conducted in 1972–1973 that among the thirty developmentally disabled persons in their investigation who were living in the community, many seemed to have learned to do without work rather nicely, while their dominating interests were recreation, hobbies, leisure, good times, friends, and family (Edgerton and Bercovici, 1974). Additional research in this area is needed. Perhaps the significance of reimburseable work is not the same for all developmentally disabled persons; it may be more appropriate to provide alternatives—yet to be described—for the developmentally disabled population to make their contribution within the creative arts. Some opportunities have been made available in a few areas of the country, with very satisfying results.

In Oakland County, Michigan, the Association for Retarded Citizens (ARC) has sponsored the Conservatory of Performing Arts. This service supplements regular school programs for children and provides opportunities for children and adults to develop artistic ability in visual arts, drama, creative dance, ballet, social folk dance, mime, and musical instrumentation. The same ARC annually sponsors the Michigan Performing Arts Talent Competition which attracts 400–500 observers while awards are given for superior performances. Such programs provide opportunities for society's enrichment as well as individual self-fulfillment.

> As an artist and as a teacher, I know that the art of the mentally retarded can be exhilarating and rewarding to the teacher, to the retarded, and to the general public . . . many of the works produced stand as art in their own right. The vigor, the use of color, the organization, and the intensity of feeling are a worthwhile contribution to our society (Ludins-Katz, 1972).

Alternative living arrangements have been developed in recent years which permit developmentally disabled adults to move toward independence in the least restrictive environment that can be provided. "Application of present knowledge makes life in normal community situations possible for the vast majority of retarded children and adults without imposing undue hardship on their families, their neighbors or those who care for them. Resort to life in institutions is less and less necessary and will probably disappear in another 25 to 50 years" (President's Committee on Mental Retardation, 1976). Innovative approaches are being tried that will provide increasingly independent living in accommodations that are acceptable to the developmentally disabled adult. Many developmentally disabled adults live in their own apartments with minimal support or assistance. Group homes in the community—ideally composed of no more than twelve residents—are successfully operating in many areas. Public acceptance of these residents is growing as it becomes evident that they can contribute to community life.

Support for the development of alternative living arrangements has been provided through different funding mechanisms. In 1971, a mechanism for low cost financing of construction of new low income housing for mentally retarded adults was designed under the Michigan State Housing Development Authority, and then made possible through the Federal Housing Act. Citizen groups formed nonprofit housing corporations in order to sponsor these homes.

Efforts continue to develop better housing for developmentally disabled adults. The stereotypical view of the developmentally disabled adult as a threat is often reflected in zoning ordinances which have prohibited the integration of this segment of the population into community life. Statutory changes have occurred in some states that no longer permit this particular infringement on the right to adequate housing.

Litigation establishing the rights of developmentally disabled citizens has contributed in many different ways to the ability of the adult to move toward self-fulfillment. Continued emphasis is anticipated through legal action on establishing and clarifying those rights. In 1971, the United Nations Declaration on the Rights of Mentally Retarded Persons was widely distributed. Throughout the 1970s, litigation has taken place firmly establishing certain specific rights. Among the most significant are the right to treatment in the least restrictive environment, the right to payment for work, the right to equal educational opportunity.

One of the most important developments that is supportive of the move toward self-fulfillment is the citizen advocacy program. The Citizen Advocacy Project, sponsored by the National Association for Retarded Citizens and funded by the Bureau of Education for the Handicapped, the National Institute of Mental Health, and the Rehabilitation Services Administration of the U.S. Department of Health, Education, and Welfare, was initiated in 1972. One of the

goals of the Project was to evolve standarized training materials so
that local and state advocacy offices could be set up by ARC's, advocates could be recruited and trained, potential proteges could be
identified, and these two groups could be matched on a one-to-one
basis. State ARC's have responded with the development of programs
of different sizes and degrees of success.

Citizen advocacy as defined by the NARC Project for mentally
retarded persons is basically a one-to-one relationship between a capable volunteer ("advocate") and a mentally retarded person ("protege") in which the advocate defends the rights and interests of the
protege and provides practical or emotional reinforcement (or a combination of both) for him. All of this occurs within the framework of a
structured advocacy system. Ideally, every developmentally disabled
adult should have an advocate. Practically, the greatest need seems to
be for those developmentally disabled adults who are leaving the institutional setting to live on an independent or semi-independent basis in
the community, those residing in institutions on a short term or long
term basis, and those of all ages and functioning levels who always
resided in the community. The relationship between the protege and
the advocate is a mutually beneficial one. The advocate's loyalty is
always to his protege. He is the friend of the protege, and he is his
mentor. One of his most important functions may be aggressive pur-
sual of services to which the protege is entitled; confrontation with
service providers is not uncommon. Another important function may
be assisting the protege to the full implementation of his rights and
responsibilities. The support and understanding of a good advocate
can be invaluable to the protege, and can be the significant factors in
the determination of successful community living.

The consideration of marriage and/or parenthood is an
important factor in the self-fulfillment of all human beings. The
President's Committee on Mental Retardation (1976) has expressed
their views related to the right of the mentally retarded to marry, and
to bear children. They believe in the following:

1. the right to be free from restrictions on the sanction to marry
2. the right to be free from involuntary sterilization
3. the right to equal access to voluntary sterilization
4. the right to procreate, nurture, and rear children.

These rights are built upon the belief that every developmentally
disabled person, as every other citizen, is presumed to be competent
and that the developmentally disabled adult must be presumed able to

make informed decisions when pertinent facts are presented in such a way that they can be understood.

As persons with developmental disabilities are able to establish their independence, they are able to successfully cope with the demands of intimacy, and the opportunity to experience it cannot be denied. The development of the intimate relationship is a very important developmental task, necessary to the process of self-actualization. It has been suggested that profoundly handicapped individuals experience their most intimate relationships with the mother or mother surrogate, a relationship not usually viewed as a sexual one.

The sexually well-adjusted moderately and mildly developmentally disabled adult will be able to successfully experience that intimate relationship through marriage. Supportive assistance can be provided. Planned group sessions for those thinking about marriage have been helpful in addressing the problems that might be anticipated. Assistance in learning the appropriate social roles, including dating, has been provided in the group meetings, or on an individual basis. Learning about sexual intercourse and childbirth has been possible in these kinds of groups. The use of contraceptives can be taught, providing facts for individual decision making in this matter.

Continued support for the married couple has been provided through the advocacy program and through community agency services. It has been suggested that sheltered living arrangements could be provided for some married couples who are unable to live independently. Minimal supervision could be provided in such settings that would be helpful in preventing the development of stressful situations.

The decision to bear children is one that can only be made with information available to the prospective parents so that their decision reflects their understanding of the responsibility involved. The fact that developmental disability is present does not preclude the possibility that effective parenting can take place, particularly if continued support is offered. Blacklidge believes that success in child rearing by mildly retarded parents depends less on the degree of retardation than it does on the emotional adjustment of the parents and on the number of children that they have. She believes that sexually well-adjusted mildly retarded adults will probably be "self-supporting, marry, and have 0–2 children" (Blacklidge, 1972).

Tomorrow, then, for the developmentally disabled adult includes the promise of fulfillment as an adult. It is realistic to expect that mildly and moderately disabled adults will be able to achieve some degree of independence, limited only by their disability. It is realistic to expect that financial independence is possible, probably through reimbursable work either in competitive employment or in a sheltered workshop experience. Most mildly and moderately developmentally disabled adults have choices about living arrangements away from the parental home. Such choices include group living arrangements with varying degrees of supervision as well as unsupervised apartment living. It is certain that social and physical integration into the community can be expected. Mildly and moderately developmentally disabled adults may choose marriage as one way of experiencing an intimate relationship. The decision to have children is one that can be made with the assistance of professionals and nonprofessionals able to assist in helping the prospective parents to assess their ability to care for the children.

The more severely developmentally disabled adult can also expect to live in the community in a group home, a foster home, or his family's home—and to be physically and socially integrated into community life, to whatever degree his disability permits. When the disability is such that a sheltered workshop experience is not feasible, enrollment in a community activity center provides the opportunity for the development of greater skills in the activities of daily living and the promotion of social adaptation. Often this type of service is available in the community in close conjunction with the community sheltered workshop. As the developmentally disabled adult acquires social skills and skill in the activities of daily living, it is often possible to arrange for transfer to the sheltered workshop.

Every developmentally disabled adult can expect health care in the community where he lives as a part of society's response to his need. Personal health services through the public health system in the community is available to him, in accordance with statutory provisions. Medical services provided through in-patient and out-patient facilities in the community are available to him. Reimbursement is often possible through Medicaid, Medicare, or health insurance benefits. Nursing service within the health care system has the potential for important contribution. Nurses can play a major role in health teaching of developmentally disabled adults, and the persons who have some responsibility for their care in nursing homes, foster homes and group homes. Nurses can provide primary care to those developmentally disabled adults who have chronic physical and emotional problems. Nurses are able to provide health counseling in groups or on an individual basis to developmentally disabled adults.

Significant contributions are being made by nurses, particularly as related to sexual activity, contraception, and procreation. And, of course, nurses are significant contributors to acute care and treatment in in-patient and out-patient settings.

Physical and social integration into community life includes having the opportunity for recreational and social activity as it occurs in the community. Regardless of the kind of housing being provided for the developmentally disabled adult, or his degree of disability, he is expected to take part in the recreational and social life of his particular community. It is here that the advocate can function very effectively. By demonstrating his friendship for the protege, and assisting him to pursue recreational and social activity that appeals to him, he serves as a model for others in the community.

Every developmentally disabled adult, who so desires, should be able to have the services of an advocate to assist him in a very personal way with his life experiences.

The future for the developmentally disabled adult is filled with promise, but it is dependent upon the acceptance by each person in our society of a personal responsibility to contribute to the development of humanistic values that can guide our actions.

## REFERENCES CITED

Blacklidge, V. 1972. What is Successful Sexual Adjustment for the Mentally Retarded? In: E. Katz (ed.), Mental health Services for the Mentally Retarded, pp. 194–211. Charles C Thomas, Springfield, Ill.

Edgerton, R. B., and Bercovici, S. M. 1976. The cloak of competence: years later. Am. J. Ment. Defic. 80(5):485–497.

Ludins-Katz, F. 1972. Creative Art Expression of the Mentally Retarded. In: E. Katz (ed.), Mental health Services for the Mentally Retarded, pp. 134–143. Charles C Thomas, Springfield, Ill.

Maslow, A. H. 1962. Some Basic Propositions of a Growth and Self-Actualization Psychology. In: Perceiving, Behaving, Becoming. Association for Supervision and Curriculum Development, National Education Association. Washington, D.C.

Meyer, Virginia R. 1973. The psychology of the young adult. Nursing Clin. N. Am. 8(1):5–14.

National Association for Retarded Citizens. 1974. Avenues to Change, Book I. NARC, Arlington, Tex.

Mental Retardation: Century of Decision. 1976. President's Committee on Mental Retardation. U.S. Government Printing Office, Washington, D.C.

President's Committee on Mental Retardation. 1975. Mental Retardation: The Known and the Unknown. U.S. Government Printing Office, Washington, D.C.

President's Committee on Mental Retardation. 1976. Mental Retardation: Century of Decision. U.S. Government Printing Office, Washington, D.C.

# INDEX

Adolescence
  assuring adequate nutrition
    throughout, 142
  developmental tasks of, 61–62
  disability, the law, and, 213–232
  as family crisis period, 81
  nutrient requirements translated into
    food needs in, 151–152
  nutrition and nutrition education
    needs in, 139–172
  nutritional requirements during,
    143–155
  possible nutritional deficiencies in,
    148
Adolescent
  in the community, 91–101
  with developmental disability, 57–58
  factors affecting nutritional
    requirements, 152–153
  and the family, 75–90
  level of cognition and expectations
    for, 63–67
  mildly retarded, educational and
    vocational expectations, 64
  moderately retarded, educational
    and vocational expectations,
    64–65
  nurses' responsibility for, 17–48
  and parents, 78–79
Adolescent period, developmental
    disability during, 6–7
Advocacy, 38–42
  preventive, and the nurse, 214–216
Assessment
  behavioral, 70
  educational and vocational, 109–115
  as first step in nursing process,
    18–32
  intellectual, 67–68
  perceptual motor, 68
  personality, 69–70
  psychological, 67–70
  in sexual counseling of
    developmentally disabled,
    192–196
  vocational, 68

Assistance for developmentally
    disabled, 216–218
Association for Retarded Citizens, 13

Behavior therapy, 72–73
  uses for, 72

Calcium requirements in adolescence,
    148–149
Calories, needs of adolescents,
    144–146
Caries, dental, 120–121
Case management of developmentally
    disabled adolescents, 37–38
Cognition, level of, 63–67
Cognitive function, determining level
    of, 63
Community
  adolescent in the, 91–101
  program for deinstitutionalization of
    developmentally disabled,
    96–97

Deinstitutionalization, 92–97
  community education, 100
  community program, 96–97
  identification process, 96
  interagency communication, 98–99
  job placement, 96
  obstacles to community service
    delivery, 97–98
  role of the institution staff, 99–100
  support services, 97
  transition process, 96
Dental needs
  of adolescents, 119–138
  dental appointments, 132–136
  financial considerations, 131–132
  referral to professionals, 130–131
  transportation and office
    accessibility, 132

Development
    historical changes in, in United
        States, 49–50
    normal adolescent, 61–62
    periods of rapid growth, 49
    physical, 49–60
Developmental disability: *see*
        Disability, developmental
Direction, verbal, in vocational
        training, 177
Disability
    adolescence, the law, and, 213–232
    developmental
        adolescent with, 57–58
        prevalence of, 2–6
Disabled, developmentally
    assistance and bill of rights, 216–219
    community service, needs of, 97
    current status of vocational
        education and rehabilitation
        programs, 177–183
    deinstitutionalization, 92–97
    education, 219–220
    employment, 220–223
    implications of behavior therapy for,
        73
    marital relationships for adult,
        66–67
    production capacity of, 174–175
    psychosocial development of, 62
    public policy for, 8–15
    residential living alternatives, 92
    rights of, 191–192
    sex education, 187–211
    sexuality of, 188–191
    use of projective tests with, 69–70
    vocational needs of, 173–185


Education
    for developmentally disabled,
        219–220
    nutrition
        assessment and planning of needs
            in, 159–170
        needs in adolescents, 139–172
    prevocational, 108
    programming, 106–108

    special, needs for, 103–118
    vocational, 181–183
Education for All Handicapped
        Children Act (P.L. 94-142),
        14, 215, 223
Employment
    of developmentally disabled,
        220–223
    state statutes regarding, 226–232
Endocrinology of puberty, 50
Expectations for developmentally
        disabled adolescents, 63–67


Family
    adolescent and the, 75–90
    problems, 80–81
    professional approaches, 87–88
    service needs, 84–85
    services for, 83–87
Fat, distribution of muscle and, 51–52
Fulfillment as adult, 233–243
Functional analysis in assessment of
        adolescent, 20–23


Growth
    at adolescence, 141–143
    historical changes in, in United
        States, 49–50
    linear, 50–51
    periods of rapid, 49
    stage of, and nutritional needs,
        141–142


Health maintenance in nursing of
        adolescents, 32–33
Heart disease, fat intake and
        development of, 148
Home visits in nursing of adolescents,
        23–24
    alternatives to, 25–26
Home Visit Guide, Siantz/Austin
        Illustrated System (SAIS),
        24–30


Intake, in assessment of adolescent,
        18–20

Intelligence testing, criticism of, 64
Interdisciplinary approaches to
    nursing of adolescents, 33–34
Intervention, therapeutic, 70–73
Iron requirements in adolescence,
    149–150

Job placement as step in
    deinstitutionalization of
    developmentally disabled, 96

Law, adolescence, disability, and,
    213–232
Legislation for handicapped, 12–14

Marriage among developmentally
    disabled adults, 66–67
Maturation, sexual, 54–57
Modeling in vocational training, 176
Muscle, distribution of fat and, 51–52

National Association for Retarded
    Children (NARC), 13–14,
    239, 240
Normalization, principle of, 7–8
Nurse
    formulation of treatment goals,
        34–36
    and preventive advocacy, 214–216
    responsibility of, in adolescence,
        17–48
Nutrition
    assuring adequate, throughout
        adolescence, 142
    and dental health, 130
    distinguishing between nutrition
        education and, 140–141
    needs in adolescence, 139–172

Obesity
    development of, in adolescence,
        146–147
    timing of growth spurt and
        development of, 142

Occlusion, 121–122
Oral hygiene, 125–129

Parenting role, 76–79
Parents
    and adolescent, 78–79
    meaning of a child to, 76–77
    responses of, to handicapped child,
        77–78
Periodontal disease, 121
Personality, assessment of, 69–70
Policy, public, for developmentally
    disabled, 8–15
Priming, physical, in vocational
    training, 176
Problems, family, 80–81
Professional feelings toward the
    disabled, 88
Programming, educational, 106–108
Protein, needs for, in adolescence,
    147–148
Psychological concepts, 61–74
Psychotherapy
    insight, group approaches to, 71–72
    insight model of, 71

Referrals to mental health
    professionals, 86
Rehabilitation, vocational, 177–181
Retarded adults, residential
    alternatives for, 65–66
Retarded, severely and profoundly,
    expectations for, 67
Rorschach test, 69

Services for families, 83–87
    strategy, 85–86
Sex education, 187–211
    curriculum, 201–207
    group vs. individual, 196
    natural approach, 196–198
    parental involvement, 201
    preventive approach, 198–199
    social learning approach, 199–201
    teaching approaches, 196–209

Sexual maturation, 54–57
Sexuality of developmentally disabled,
     188–191
Shaping in vocational training, 176
Shaping technique, use of, 72
Siantz/Austin Illustrated System
     (SAIS) Home Visit Guide,
     24–30
Sibling role, 81–83
Social Security Act of 1935, 12
Soldiers Rehabilitation Act, 12

Thematic Apperception Test, 69
Therapy, behavior, 72–73
Token economy, 73
Training procedures, vocational,
     175–177

Trauma, dental, 122
Treatment goals, formulation of,
     34–36
   inclusion of developmentally
     disabled adolescent in, 37

Vitamin D requirements in
     adolescence, 148–149
Vocational needs of developmentally
     disabled, 173–185
Vocational Rehabilitation Act, 14

Weight, change in during adolescence,
     52–54
Work study, 115–116